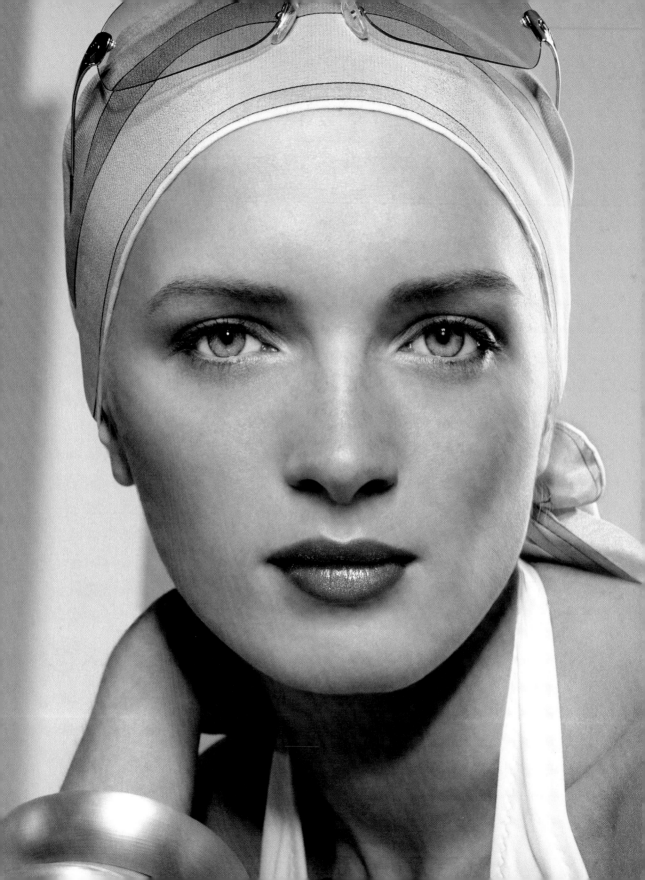

Trish McEvoy

written with KATHLEEN BOYES
design & art direction: ROBERT VALENTINE
photography: DANIELA FEDERICI,
GREG DELVES & MARTYN THOMPSON

THE POWER OF MAKEUP

LOOKING YOUR
LEVEL BEST
AT EVERY AGE

A Fireside Book
Published by Simon & Schuster
New York London Toronto Sydney

FIRESIDE
ROCKEFELLER CENTER
1230 AVENUE OF THE AMERICAS
NEW YORK, NY 10020

FIRST FIRESIDE TRADE PAPERBACK EDITION 2005

FIRESIDE AND COLOPHON ARE REGISTERED TRADEMARKS
OF SIMON & SCHUSTER, INC.

FOR INFORMATION REGARDING SPECIAL DISCOUNTS FOR BULK PURCHASES,
PLEASE CONTACT SIMON & SCHUSTER SPECIAL SALES AT 1-800-456-6798
OR BUSINESS@SIMONANDSCHUSTER.COM

DESIGNED BY ROBERT VALENTINE AND THE VALENTINE GROUP NYC

MANUFACTURED IN THE UNITED STATES OF AMERICA

10   9   8   7   6   5   4   3

THE LIBRARY OF CONGRESS HAS CATALOGED
THE HARDCOVER EDITION AS FOLLOWS
MCEVOY, TRISH.
  THE POWER OF MAKEUP : LOOKING YOUR LEVEL BEST AT EVERY AGE /
  TRISH MCEVOY WRITTEN WITH KATHLEEN BOYES
      P. CM.
  1. COSMETICS.   2. BEAUTY, PERSONAL.   3. BEAUTY CULTURE.
  I. TITLE: TRISH MCEVOY.   II. BOYES, KATHLEEN.   III. TITLE.
GT2340.M36 2003
646.7'2—DC22   2003054498

ISBN 0-7432-5036-2
    0-7432-5037-0 (Pbk)

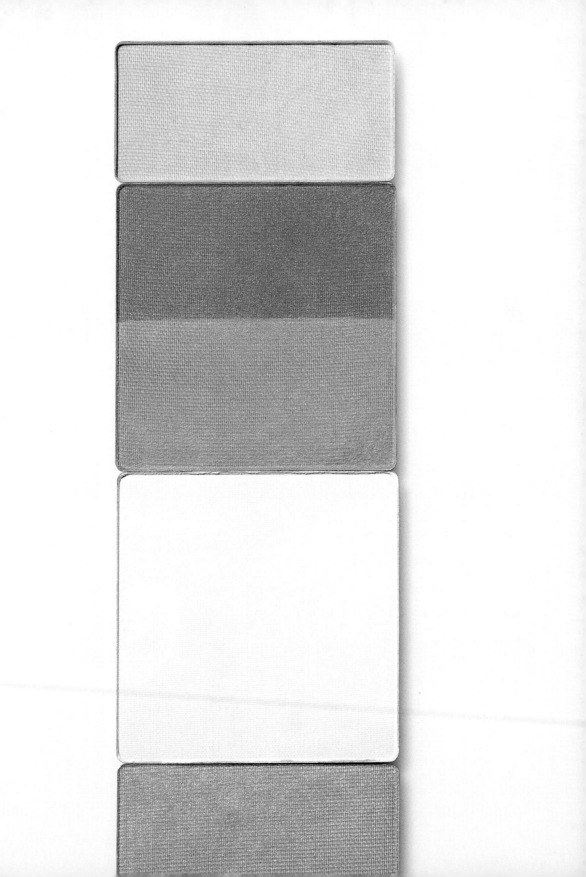

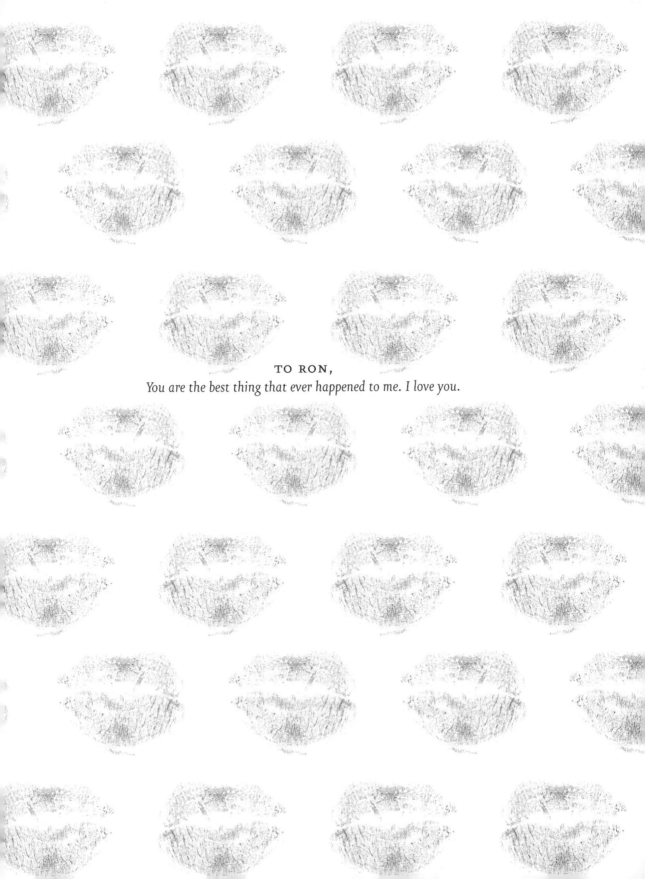

TO RON,
You are the best thing that ever happened to me. I love you.

ACKNOWLEDGMENTS

EVERY PAGE OF THIS BOOK HAS A HISTORY TO ME. IT BRINGS MY PAST INTO THE PRESENT. I BELIEVE THAT I AM TRULY BLESSED, HAVING HAD AN ANGEL ON MY SHOULDER ALL THESE YEARS. THERE ARE MANY PEOPLE WHO HAVE CONTRIBUTED TO THE PLEASURE AND SUCCESS OF MY EVERYDAY LIFE, AS WELL AS THAT OF TRISH MCEVOY LIMITED AND THE DR. RONALD SHERMAN/TRISH MCEVOY SKINCARE CENTER. I AM FORTUNATE TO HAVE ENCOUNTERED SO MANY GENEROUS INDIVIDUALS. THERE ARE CERTAIN PEOPLE WHO MUST BE MENTIONED BY NAME FOR THEIR INFLUENCE AND HELP. AT THE END OF THE DAY, LIFE ISN'T ABOUT WHAT YOU DO, BUT WHO YOU'RE LUCKY ENOUGH DO IT WITH. HERE ARE SOME OF MY EARTHLY ANGELS I WISH TO THANK.

A special thank-you to the legendary Esther Newberg, my agent at ICM who made this book happen, and to your assistants, Chris Bauch and Andy Barzvi. Thank you to my pal Judy Licht for sending me to Esther—Judy, this book may have not happened without you.

Thank you, Mark Gompertz at Simon & Schuster, for sealing the deal, and thank you, Trish Todd, my wonderful editor, for letting me do it my way and for not panicking when we needed a few extra days of photography or wanted to review the cover for the umpteenth time. Thank you to Jennifer Love, Nancy Clements, and Brett Valley for your help in turning *The Power of Makeup* into a book. Thank you to Chris Lloreda, Marcia Burch, Laurie Cotumaccio, and Sue Fleming for all the help in organizing the PR and marketing efforts.

To Kathleen Boyes, who allowed my words to take on life and for the many phone calls, faxes, e-mails, and meetings. My voice would not have come alive without your wonderful writing style. I had the great fortune of becoming your friend. You're a dream.

I've been a great admirer of designer Robert Valentine's work and was thrilled to have the opportunity to collaborate with him. Robert, I knew that with your impeccable taste and style, you'd realize my vision, and you have done so beautifully. Working with you was as much fun as it was an education. I so enjoyed the process and know we will go on to a lifetime of friendship and projects together. Thanks also to Robert's fabulous staff: Alison Kist, Brandon Jameson, Judy Minn, Ellen Elfering, and Stephen Johnson.

For the photographs, thank you, Daniela Federici, for your elegant, polished style and unfailing eye. You worked like a trouper from dawn till dusk, knowing just the right thing to say and do to achieve such exquisite images. I also thank your team, Mo Saito and Patrick Brangan from Mercury Artist Group. A special thanks to Michel Arnaud for my portrait. Thank you, Martyn Thompson and assistant Hamish Fraser, from Marek & Associates whose photo made me want to travel, and Greg Delves and assistants Tim Bell, Simon Burstell, and Mitchell Kawakami from Judy Casey Inc., who made my products look like the objects of desire I consider them to be.

Thank you, Kim Handley, George Productions, and Jeffrey Gardner, her assistant, who made production so easy. Thank you to Gemal from Sally Harlor, who does hair magic in fifteen minutes, and Sara Gore Reeves and her team, Brent Crossman, Lindsey Brush, and Cinthia Boni, who could style and dress anyone at a moment's notice. Thank you, Noemi Bonazzi, Lisa Lee, and Dominique Baynes for props. Thank you, Steve Willis, for the fabulous casting.

I thank the beautiful faces that adorn these pages: Valeria Avdeyeva from Elite, whose natural glamour and sweetness will take her far; Sarah Irvine from Wilhelmina; Chris Mosier of Ford Models; and Nanda Hampe of Next, who never complained when it was 40 degrees and she had to stand in a wet sarong. It was also a joy to work with Johanna Martensson of Wilhelmina, Cindy Joseph of Ford, and Kimanee Wilson of Elite.

Joanne Pigozzi and Geri Emmett. What can I say? You are my left and right hands in all that I do. My love and respect for you is endless. I thank you with all my heart for the memories, the smart work, the great ideas, the perfect executions, the many laughs we share. This is our life, and together we will make our future dreams come true. I look forward to it.

Thank you, Kitty Pankratz, who every day looks for beauty and who makes each day more beautiful for everyone, especially for me. The best traveling partner in the world, your creativity, innate style, and great heart are apparent in everything you touch.

I thank our outstanding team at The Dr. Ronald Sherman/Trish McEvoy Skincare Center in New York City—Robin Carter, Regina Palminteri, Carla Plundeke, Jill Caputo, Adele Genovese, Sheryl Eriksson, Natalie Govert, Kim Govert, Liliana Mina, Mia Veresmortean, Michelle McCall, and of course Dolores Espinal.

To our regional managers, past and present, who deliver my vision nationwide and the Trish McEvoy Makeup Artists across the country, I thank you for teaching our customers how to put on our makeup in an organized fashion. You represent the heart and soul of what we do.

Then there is the New Jersey team, who handle the day-to-day operations of Trish McEvoy, Limited. Rob Leonardo, thank you for coming into my company and instantly making a difference. Mikey Primelo, thank you for being there when I needed you most; you are a dear friend. Sheila Henry Park, Sarah Caban and Leslie Lang, Dina Bruce, Betsy Rodriguez, Mike Lambiaso, Marjan Hamzelou, Karen Iannaci, Lorraine Szabo, Monette Vuong, I thank you for your dedication and can-do spirit. I thank Steve Schweighofer for his immediate impact on our distribution center, as well as our distribution center staff, who are responsible for getting us out there, including fulfilling thousands of last-minute orders. And I must thank Mayra Vitale and Pam Bovell for setting things straight so many years ago.

And thank you. Gloria Gregurovich, for being the brilliant designer that you are.

My stylish mother, Ursula, was such an enormous influence in my life in terms of fashion and beauty and showed me the drive you need to make something out of nothing. You were my role model in so many ways. I also thank my sister, Romy, who has such a carefree spirit, and her children, Nadia and Cyan, whom I adore. Dominique, you're always in my heart.

Because we shared so many wonderful memories my late in-laws, Sidell and Phill, will always have a special place in my heart . . . not a day goes by that I don't think of you both. You set wonderful examples of true family values that I see followed every day by Pam and Ed, who display such warmth and caring for their children, Jordan and Marcie, and Jason and Trisha. The same is true of Spencer and Sue and their children, Sabrina and Robert, and Christine and Kelly. The loving example continues right on down to all your precious great-grandchildren.

Ester and Michael Pantzer and their children Karen and Jessica, you are dear to my heart, and I consider you family.

Thank you, Argentina Ricardo, Augusto C. Ricardo, and Delores Ramos, for waking me every day with coffee and a smile and for making the domestic side of my life run smoothly. You take great care of me, and it is deeply appreciated.

I want to thank the clients who believed in me way back when, as I traveled with trunks of makeup and skin care products to cities throughout the United States, long before stores happened in my life.

I want to hug all those early clients who came to the Dr. Ronald Sherman/Trish McEvoy Skincare Center in its infancy and made it a way of life, and a very special hug to you, Connie Cook.

Thank you to all the beauty editors over the years who shared the excitement, many of whom have become close friends.

Thank you, Wendy Whitworth, for a great friendship I can count on. Elaine Miller, whether you're in New York or Washington, you always come through. The same is true of you, Betsy McDonald from Atlanta; thank you. And thank you, Jane Rosenthal, another terrific friend who has graced this book with her kind words.

Thank you, Vincent Roppatte, of the Elizabeth Arden Salon; John Barrett and your fabulous team, and Ania for always making it a good hair day.

To dear Ed Burstell of Henri Bendel, a man whose instincts and vision I so respect and admire. I thank you for your friendship and committed support. I also thank Laura Saio and Louise Evans.

To Deborah Walters at Saks Fifth Avenue, you manage a big business and always remain a lady. You truly are a special woman who has always been there for us; thank you and your team, including Kate Oldham, Pam Thomas, Wendy Godfriend Marla Glastein, and Nathan Barnhill.

To the creative Dale Crichton of Nordstrom, who believed in us from the beginning, thank you and your team of true ladies, including Laura Hubbard, Peggy Mansur, Nootsie McNabb, and Andrea Nakagaki.

Thank you to those at Neiman Marcus: Burt Tansky, Neva Hall, Leslie Faust, Hazel Wyatt, Muriel McNatt, as well as Jim Gold, my new best friend. You all bravely keep pushing the envelope, and I admire you so.

Thank you, Bergdorf Goodman's Murial Gonzalas, Pat Saxbe, and Jennifer Miles, who make Fifth Avenue just a little more special.

To Bloomingdale's Michael Gould, Francine Klein, Nancy Feldman, and Gail Perfetto, who opened the doors to Federated for me. Thank you for the magic you create every day.

Thank you, Patrick Hanley and Daniella Rinaldi of Harvey Nichols, for bringing us to the other side of the ocean. I can't forget Howard Koch from Parisian, one of the first who helped us reach southern belles, nor Irene Price and Larry Williams at Jacobson's, also among the early believers

I remain ever grateful to the small, special boutiques across America that are a treat for the Trish McEvoy clients to visit each and every day.

This book is a culmination of a life and career of making up thousands of women's faces. Thank you all for your friendship and the many laughs along the way.

FOREWORD

EVERY WOMAN LOVES MAKEUP.

As a little girl, I was always fascinated by the mysterious products that my cousin
Estelle sold behind the counter at our local department store in Providence.
I just knew that whatever magic lay in those compacts and tubes was exactly what
I needed to become a new me! I hoarded as many samples as I could beg
my cousin to give me and then spent hours hiding in the bathroom and playing
with my new grown-up toys.

A few years ago, I realized that I was still applying my makeup the same way
I did in seventh grade, when cousin Estelle showed me how to shmear a
"little something" on my cheeks. I was practically using the same products.
I called my friend Elizabeth Saltzman with my beauty 911, and she
sent me straight to Trish McEvoy.

At the beginning of my appointment, Trish asked how she could help.
I said, "I'm turning forty, I have a two-year-old daughter, a full-time job, and I really
need a vacation but I'm about to start production on a film and have zero time
to go anywhere. Help!" I remember thinking there is no way that kind of help comes
in a bottle. Then Trish went to work. Ten minutes later, I looked in the mirror
and staring back was a seemingly rested me—but me fresh off the plane from
a tropical island. Suddenly my face was sun kissed, I looked relaxed, and I couldn't
imagine where she put those circles I kept under my eyes.

Trish and I became friendly after that first session. From the beginning, what I loved about Trish was how she got my lifestyle; I'm still that little girl wanting to play with the pretty products, but I don't have all that time to spend locked in the bathroom anymore. Trish taught me how to fit a beauty regimen into my life in a way that is artful and professional and takes under ten minutes as I'm racing out of the house at 7:45 A.M.

Trish never settles; her versatile system changes to fit my life. She listens to her clients and customizes her products for all our needs. Trish's products look so enticing that you absolutely need to hold, touch, and use these beautiful little packages. Trish is always growing with her product so that we can grow with her product, too.

Makeup transforms us. Trish has helped me put my best foot—er, face —forward and present to the world a well-rested, vacationed me, no matter how long it has been since I've had a full eight hours sleep. And all in seven minutes! Or five . . . or three . . .

Whether you know Trish personally or you end up getting to know her makeup line, you discover how much she loves what she does. She understands that women wear many faces every day for the many facets of their lives. She appreciates a woman's life, and she celebrates it.

JANE ROSENTHAL
Cofounder/producer Tribeca Productions

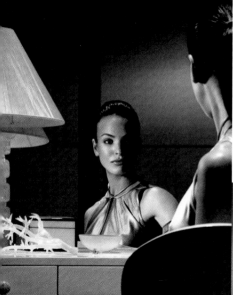
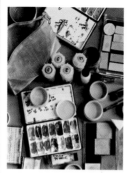
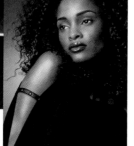
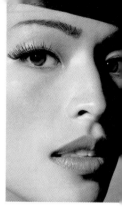
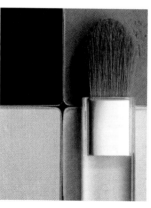
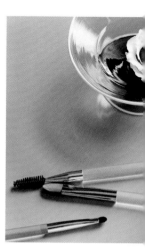
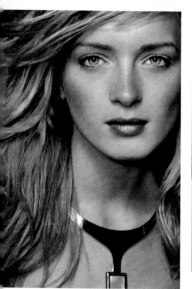
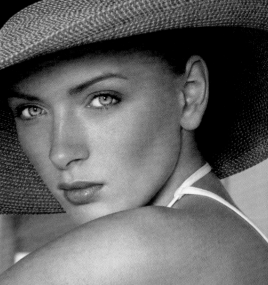
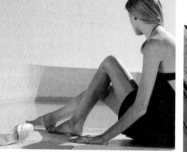
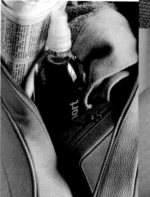

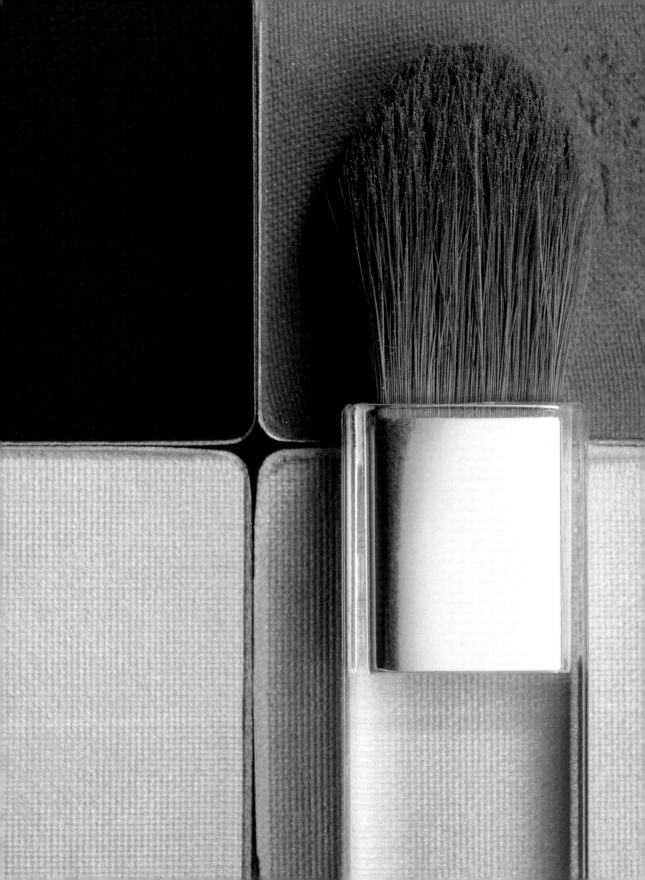

A PASSION FOR MAKEUP: *A Philosophy of Beauty*

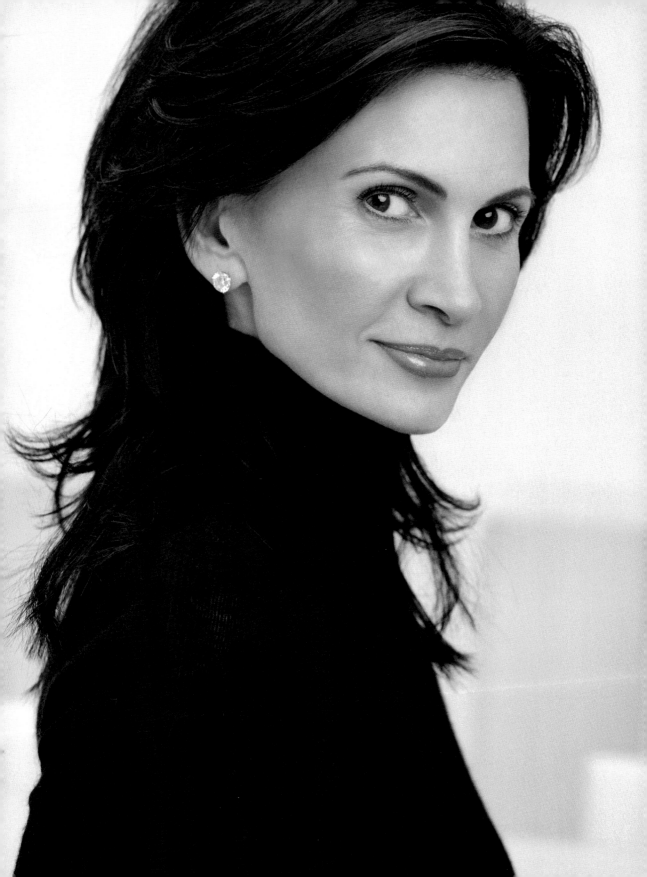

I love the power and wonder of makeup. Absolutely adore it. There is simply nothing that is more transforming or more glamorizing. Makeup is an instant lift and, on certain days, a real lifesaver. Makeup has also made me dear friends with so many women, yet another reason I love what I do. Nothing bonds women faster than a shared tip, a great new color, or some really good advice. The minute a woman sits in my chair, I know that we'll soon be chatting up a storm and laughing. What's not to love about makeup?

THIS BOOK IS DESIGNED TO BE YOUR OWN MAKEUP CONSULTATION. IF YOU'RE LIKE MANY OF THE WOMEN I'VE CONSULTED WITH OVER THE YEARS, YOU'RE PROBABLY EXCITED YET A BIT INTIMIDATED BY THE PROSPECT OF A MAKEUP CONSULTATION. ABOUT THE INTIMIDATED PART, LET ME PUT YOUR MIND AT EASE RIGHT AWAY. MAKEUP IS NOT SOME KIND OF EXCLUSIVE, RAREFIED ART.

Makeup is something everyone can master. Yes, I am a makeup artist, and my eye is better trained, my hand a little more practiced, but that's because I've been at the trial and error thing a lot longer than you have. I am completely self-taught, and I consider myself to be still learning. I experiment, I play, and I'm open to trying anything at least once.

Have an open mind. Follow my advice and you will have a better understanding of makeup and makeup products. That knowledge will give you confidence about the makeup you choose to wear and how you apply it. Most of all, I hope to show you how much fun you can have along the way. Makeup is all about possibility, the pleasure of discovery, the adventure of creating your individual look.

On an emotional level, makeup is an instant pick-me-up. When a woman comes to me, she's eager to learn. I derive tremendous enjoyment and satisfaction from watching her do it all on her own. I set out to make my client feel better about herself. If you look good, you feel good: it's really that simple and that fundamental. By the time you finish this book, I want you to feel that makeup is your friend.

One of the many other reasons I love makeup is that I truly enjoy the time I spend applying it. My makeup application is the one time of the day that I give myself for sheer luxury. Because we're all so busy, those few minutes can give you the time to collect yourself as you prepare for the day (or evening). Makeup can provide the kind of private time in which not only do you transform your look, but you transform your mood and get ready to face the day.

When I was a child, I used to spend hours meticulously coloring in coloring books. I discovered that if you pressed harder on the crayon, the line was more defined. If you pressed lighter, the effect was softer. Oh, how I strove to get each picture perfect! And that's really how good makeup happens . . . with the patience to blend properly, and then blend some more. Looking your best is doable. It's just a matter of knowing your style, organizing yourself, and learning the techniques that truly make a world of difference.

I will walk you through every step, telling you exactly what you need to know, what works and what doesn't. Each makeup product is a building block, applied step by step, Level by Level (a concept of mine we'll soon explore at length). We'll make sure you master the basics before you move on to anything more advanced.

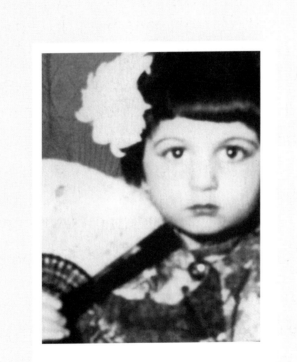

I'VE PUT A LOT OF TIME AND THOUGHT INTO MAKING MAKEUP EASY. EASY IS KEY, BECAUSE IF SOMETHING IS DIFFICULT, I WON'T DO IT, AND I SUSPECT YOU WON'T EITHER. I'VE DEVELOPED AND PATENTED THE PLANNER—A BINDER OF MAKEUP—THE SOLE PURPOSE OF WHICH IS TO EDIT AND ORGANIZE YOUR MAKEUP AND TOOLS FOR USE AT HOME AND ON THE ROAD. THERE'S NO REASON TO CARRY EVERY PRODUCT YOU OWN EVERYWHERE YOU GO (UNLESS YOU WANT TO, OF COURSE, AND SOME WOMEN DO). NOR SHOULD YOU BE RUMMAGING AROUND AT THE BOTTOM OF A BAG FOR A LIPSTICK OR WONDERING WHERE YOU LAST LEFT YOUR FAVORITE BLUSH. IT'S GREAT TO HAVE ALL YOUR MAKEUP IN ONE PLACE. THAT WAY YOU HAVE EXACTLY THE PRODUCTS YOU NEED AT YOUR FINGER-TIPS EXACTLY WHEN YOU NEED THEM. EDITING YOUR MAKEUP IS SIMPLE, AND I'LL TEACH YOU HOW TO DO IT.

I've also come up with a system of application that I know works. I have good reasons why you should apply products in a certain order, and I will share them all with you. I want you to enjoy yourself, but I also want you to get it right, so that by the time you leave the makeup mirror, you have the confidence to forget about it.

Confidence is the most flattering thing in the world. The secret to achieving confidence is to have peace of mind and be comfortable in your own skin. That's why I'm here—not to reinvent your personal style, just to enhance it. You've spent a lifetime cultivating the way you live and dress, and I respect that. I want you to try new ideas, fresh colors, and great techniques, but only within your comfort zone. You have to feel at home in your face, and your face has to complement your total look, including what you wear. My goal is to help you look your absolute Level best and have a good time in the process.

I want you to see that good makeup is an exciting reality you can achieve. It can make you look younger, fresher, and more glamorous. Makeup can be magical. I'm an optimistic realist. I want you to stop looking at what's wrong with your looks and focus on what's right. We'll magnify the positive and minimize the negative. I'm a firm believer that it's all in your attitude. A positive spirit can accomplish anything it sets out to. I've seen it happen firsthand, starting with three special women in my life.

A LEGACY OF GLAMOUR

LET ME TELL YOU ABOUT THREE OF THE GREATEST FEMALE INFLUENCES
IN MY LIFE. IN THEIR OWN SEPARATE WAYS, EACH WOMAN WAS OBSESSED WITH
BEAUTY YET USED HER BRAIN AND DRIVE TO MAKE BEAUTY WORK FOR HER.

For the first five years of my life, I lived with my grandparents in Berlin. My grandmother was a strong, dynamic woman who owned and operated a perfumery. There I would play with the beautiful bottles and jars and watch her help clients. Given the day and age, it wasn't easy for a woman to be an entrepreneur. My grandmother encouraged me to play, dress up, express myself, and make believe. I also experienced the magic of scent. I was fortunate to have spent my formative years with this extraordinary woman.

When I was five, my mother took me and my sister to live in France. Our life in Versailles was different and difficult, but my mother always strove to look her best, with her special purse and whatever fashion piece of the moment she could afford. Style was important to my mother. She was a glamorous woman with a sense of fantasy. I can remember being mesmerized while I watched her apply makeup, spray on perfume, and slather on body lotion. I was twelve when she brought us to America, where we began the next chapter of our lives, in Georgia.

As I look back, I can't help but admire how gutsy my mother was to leave her culture, kids in tow, and begin anew. Blessed with a can-do attitude, she became successfully self-employed selling exercise machines. (I'm sure her customers took one look at her svelte figure and bought a machine on the spot.) I still think of my mother as a glamorous movie star. Now in her seventies, she still looks fabulous, still lives in Georgia, and when she goes out driving in her little old white convertible, she wears leather driving gloves and just the right amount of makeup for her style.

The third influential woman in my life is my mother-in-law. She was a homemaker who poured all her energies into her marriage, two sons, and daughter. My mother-in-law, now in her mid-nineties, is as elegant as she is strong. A fabulously stylish woman, she is always done from head to toe, starting with her salon-coiffed hair and beautifully tailored clothes. She tells it to you straight, pulling no punches, yet she's always a lady about it. You have to admire such a spirited, truly beautiful woman.

What I've learned from all of these women is that a sense of elegance is essential. When my mother had tough times, it would have been easy for her not to care about how she looked, but she insisted on looking her best. My mother has always believed that no matter where you are or what you have, you have to have that specialness in your life that elegance brings.

MY PATH TO BEAUTY

YOU HAVE TO FIND YOUR OWN WAY IN THIS WORLD. MOVING FROM GERMANY TO FRANCE AND THEN TO AMERICA, I LEARNED HOW TO SIZE UP A SITUATION, ADAPT QUICKLY, AND STAY OPEN-MINDED. CHANGE CAN BE A GOOD THING, BUT I TURNED IT INTO A GREAT THING. I LEARNED THAT THERE'S NO REASON TO BE SCARED OF THE UNKNOWN. I ALSO DISCOVERED THAT I LOVED MEETING NEW PEOPLE.

WHEN I WAS EIGHTEEN, I MOVED TO VIRGINIA AND GOT A JOB AT A MAKEUP COUNTER IN A SPECIALTY STORE. HAVING SPENT MY YOUTH PLAYING WITH CREAMS, LOTIONS, AND COLOR, I LEARNED THE APPLICATION PART QUICKLY. I LOVED MY JOB. I IMMEDIATELY DISCOVERED THE JOY OF LISTENING TO A WOMAN'S CONCERNS AND MAKING HER FEEL BETTER BY APPLYING HER MAKEUP AND BUILD-ING UP HER CONFIDENCE. AFTER SOME TIME, THE COSMETIC COMPANY I WORKED FOR PROMOTED ME TO "VISITING MAKEUP ARTIST AND SKIN CARE SPECIALIST," SENDING ME TO OTHER STORES. THIS GAVE ME THE OPPORTUNITY TO BE ON LOCAL TELEVISION AND RADIO SHOWS, REACHING YET MORE WOMEN.

My next step was New York City. I instantly fell in love with New York, made it my home, and continued traveling to stores across the country, loving every minute of it.

Nineteen seventy-five was a very good year for me. I left corporate life and started working part-time at a trendy make-up/pharmacy store. In the evenings, I worked on test photo shoots with new photographers and young models. We were all learning our professions together. The work I did on photo shoots let me see how makeup, different textures, and techniques photographed. One of the models, Connie Cook (who went on to become one of Halston's favorites), became a close friend and started recommending my makeup and skin-care services to her friends.

During this time, I was honing my craft and experimenting with textures, colors, application, and skin care. I realized that there were many gaps in the beauty field. I had ideas about products I wanted to develop. I experimented with items available at that time, subtly tweaking them—adding yellow pigment to foundations that were too pink, sheering out foundations, and adding shimmer to lip and cheek colors.

Since you're only as good as the tools you use, I went to an art store to buy brushes and started reshaping them myself. I took the prototypes to a brush manufacturer and had six brushes made to my specifications. Not surprisingly, I'd make up someone's face, and she'd want to buy the brush on the spot because it made the application so easy. A business was born.

Everything I develop starts with a prototype—the first version of what I have in mind. Whatever the product, I have to love it and live with it. I use it over and over to know if it's truly right. I need to see how it performs and if it works with other products. For example, if it's foundation, I need to know if it layers well and how it works on the skin. If I'm developing something like sheer lip gloss, I want to make sure the tint of color, the texture, and the feel on the lips is what I envisioned. Should I be working on a skin care product, I want it to work synergistically with my system of products. I will test and retest a product until it is perfect.

My lab is wherever I am working that week—my office, my kitchen table, or my hotel room. Next to me, you will always find a million little tubes, bottles, and jars as well as the latest assortment of paint boxes full of different textures and formulas. Mind you, I never have just one project going on. I'm constantly improving existing formulas and developing new products. My business is always a work in progress, and I enjoy every minute of the fine-tuning. The final moment of satisfaction comes when I apply the product on someone else, stand back, and say, "Wow. It's just what I wanted."

MY HUSBAND, DR. RONALD SHERMAN

MY HUSBAND, RONALD SHERMAN, IS A WONDERFUL NEW YORK CITY DERMA-TOLOGIST. I'VE LEARNED A GREAT DEAL FROM HIM ABOUT WHAT CAN BE DONE FOR SKIN MEDICALLY AS WELL AS PREVENTIVELY. HE'S TAUGHT ME ABOUT IN-GREDIENTS THAT CAN TRULY MAKE A DIFFERENCE AND TREATMENTS THAT CAN DRAMATICALLY IMPROVE SKIN.

When Ron and I met in the late seventies, dermatology was focused solely on treating problem skin. Ron and I believed that making people look good and feel good involved more than that, and we joined forces. The combination of a dermatologist and a makeup artist/skin-care specialist in one office was nothing short of revolutionary. Our skin care center was one of the first to combine medical and cosmetic treatments; we educated women about their skin and their home regimens and continue to do so today. Over the years, it has given us such joy to see the many generations of patients and clients coming through our doors. We love the fact that the office at 800A always has such a family feel.

TRISH MCEVOY, LTD.

I incorporated my business when I was twenty-five years old. My brush collection, which had earned a following among professionals and clients alike, was in great demand. I immediately began adding makeup products to the collection. It was thrilling to be able to work directly with the manufacturers and lab technicians to make products to my specifications. Having a hand in a product's development is liberating. You get exactly what you want, and, on my end, it makes my work nearly effortless.

Throughout the eighties, I expanded my business, adding more makeup as well as skin care products, and working full days meeting clients at the makeup and skin center. I started thinking about the next step for my small company. To reach a wider audience, I knew I had to expand my business into retail stores. I remember placing a call to Ed Burstell at Henri Bendel and telling him I thought the time had come. He agreed!

That first year of selling makeup and educating women at Bendel was absolutely thrilling. It was 1993 and the start of my taking my cosmetic line across the United States and eventually overseas. I love traveling and meeting the people who work at my counters, and especially meeting you the customer in all the stores that carry my line, including Saks Fifth Avenue, Nordstrom, Neiman Marcus, Harvey Nichols, Bergdorf Goodman, Bloomingdale's, and Parisian, as well as many beautiful spas and makeup boutiques. As I look back and see how the business has grown over the years, it's hard to imagine that it all began with just a brush and a dream.

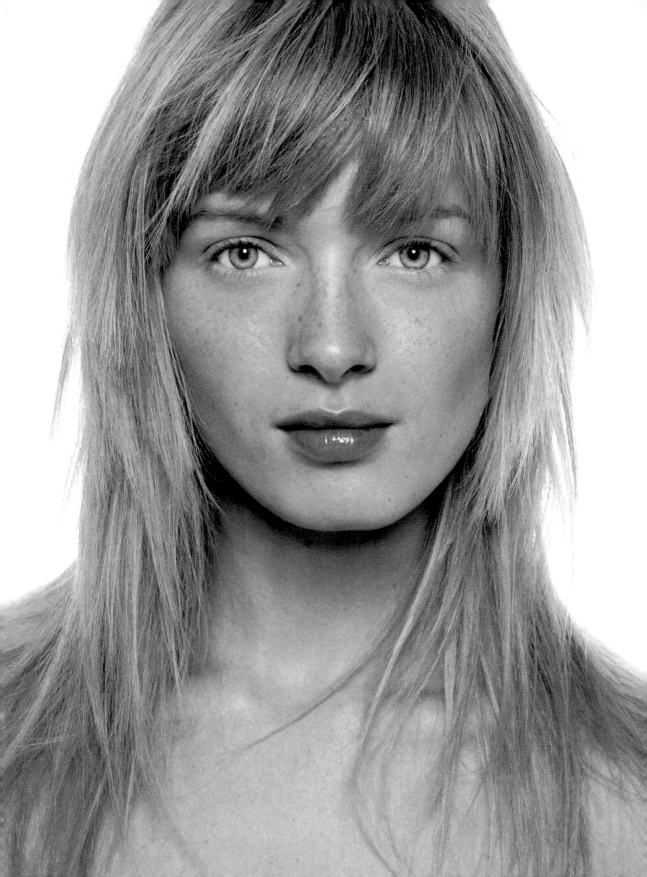

SKIN CARE: *The Absolute Essentials and Then Some*

Our skin is always changing due to age, hormones, and climate, as well as our activities. Because skin is always changing, its needs are always shifting. You'll look your best if you analyze your skin on a day-to-day, climate-to-climate basis and treat it accordingly. You want to promote a healthy radiance. I'm going to give you some good, basic guidelines that, if followed, will make a world of difference to your skin's condition now and in the future.

I'm lucky: I can learn about all the latest important medical breakthroughs in skin care from my husband, Dr. Ronald Sherman. Skin-care technology has advanced greatly, and innovations are introduced all the time. Of course, when it comes to your skin, taking a step back and being a bit conservative can pay off in the long run. You want to wait until something is truly proven safe and effective before you try it.

Today there are products and treatments that can actually enhance the appearance and texture of skin, as well as help diminish the appearance of fine lines. Both your daily skin-care routine and special treatments should support your skin's particular needs.

THE FOUR ESSENTIALS

I BELIEVE STRONGLY IN THE SYNERGY OF A FOUR-STEP
APPROACH TO BASIC SKIN CARE. THE FOUR STEPS ARE CLEANSING,
EXFOLIATING, MOISTURIZING, AND PROTECTING.

I. CLEANSING

No matter how tired or short on time you are, regular cleansing is an important part of healthy skin maintenance. Do not neglect this step! Its purpose is to remove makeup, debris, and dead skin cells.

CHOICES: *Cleansing balms, cleansing creams, cleansing washes, and cleansing bars. As a general rule, drier skins do better with creamier textures, and oilier skins do better with washes or bars.*

2. EXFOLIATING

The difference between dull skin and glowing skin is right on the surface. The most common cause of dull complexions is a decreased rate of cell turnover. Exfoliation helps the skin look its freshest by refining the surface and restoring its natural radiance. Everyone can benefit from this vital step of removing dead skin cells, which results in a smoother complexion. Exfoliation also allows better penetration of treatment products and moisturizers. Always remember to use your sunscreen in conjunction with any kind of exfoliation, because the new skin you expose is especially vulnerable. How often you exfoliate depends on how your skin looks. If your skin looks dull or if makeup catches on your skin as you apply it, you need to exfoliate. Some people make it a part of their daily skin care regimen, and others do it no more than twice a week—the minimum I would recommend.

CHOICES: *You have options here. There are different types, some that contain alpha hydroxy acids (AHAs) and beta hydroxy acids (BHAs) and some that don't. Check the label to determine what, if any, acid is included.*

MASKS AND SCRUBS:

Considered the first generation of exfoliation and still popular choices, especially when AHA or BHA is not an option because of skin sensitivity. When purchasing a scrub, look for one that contains smooth, synthetic spherical beads, which are more gentle on the skin.

AHAS AND BHAS:

Many exfoliants contain acids, which have the ability to exfoliate and smooth the skin's surface, as well as speed up the generation of new cells.

ALPHA HYDROXY ACIDS. The most common is glycolic acid, considered the most effective at improving the overall appearance of the skin since it has the smallest molecule, which allows for the deepest penetration. Glycolic acids can be irritating to extremely sensitive skin types.

BETA HYDROXY ACIDS. More commonly known as salicylic acids, BHAs are slightly milder than AHAs. They are used to target acne and clear pores as well as improve skin tone and reduce inflammation.

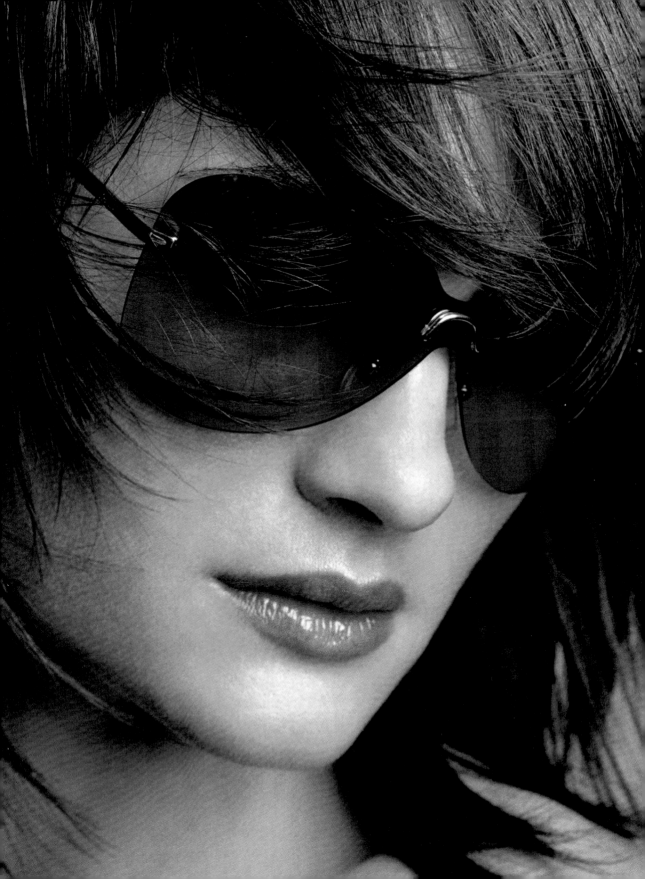

3. MOISTURIZING

Moisturizers deliver water to the skin, temporarily plump up fine lines, and smooth and soften the appearence of the skin. They also lock in the water that is already there. It's just a matter of choosing which formula is right for your skin type. Use an oil-free moisturizer if you have normal or oily skin; if you have dry skin, you can use a more enriched formula.

4. PROTECTING

This is a must! Nothing will help you avoid sun damage and wrinkles more than using a daily sunblock or sunscreen. An SPF of 15 with UVA and UVB protection should be the minimum you wear. Apply sunscreen thirty minutes before going outside.

DAILY SUN CARE. On the days when you have limited sun exposure, a moisturizer with a sunscreen is a good choice. It should have an SPF of at least 15. The great part is that it's as easy as applying a moisturizer— a true no-brainer.

OUTDOOR SUN CARE. If you know you'll be spending considerable time outside (for instance playing golf or tennis or going to the beach), step up your sun care regimen. Increase your protection factor to an SPF of 30 and remember to reapply every two hours, especially after swimming and vigorous exercise.

SENSITIVE-SKIN SUN CARE. Nonchemical sun products work by creating a physical barrier over the skin. Look for ingredients like titanium dioxide or zinc oxide. Zinc oxide, which traditionally is white and opaque, is now also available in a transparent form to give even the most sensitive skin a broad spectrum of protection.

VITAMINS AND THE SKIN

VITAMINS ARE ONE OF THE BIGGEST TRENDS IN BEAUTY AND SKIN CARE PRODUCTS. TOPICAL PRODUCTS, WHETHER SOLD OVER THE COUNTER OR BY PRESCRIPTION, CAN PROVIDE VISIBLE IMPROVEMENTS IN FINE LINES, A BRIGHTENING OF THE COMPLEXION, AND IMPROVEMENT IN TEXTURE. THE VITAMINS DISCUSSED HERE ARE ALL ANTIOXIDANTS, MEANING THAT THEY DISARM MOLECULES CALLED FREE RADICALS. FREE RADICALS ARE A BY-PRODUCT OF AN ENVIRONMENTAL IRRITANT SUCH AS SUN, SMOKE, OR POLLUTION.

VITAMIN A. When buying skin-care products, the vitamin A family is one of the best investments you can make. Years of scientific research have proved that certain Vitamin A derivatives catagorized as retinoids can significantly improve years of accumulated sun damage and can clear up acne. When shopping for a skin product with vitamin A, look for the words *retinol, retinyl acetate, retinyl linoleate,* or *retinyl palmitate.* Remember, vitamin A increases your sensitivity to the sun, so don't forget to wear your sunscreen!

RETINOIC ACID. A derivative of vitamin A, retinoic acid has the FDA's approval for treating acne and skin aging. Tretinoin, as found in prescription medications (Retin A and Renova), enhances the skin's ability to renew itself, reduces fine lines, evens out pigmentation, and smooths surface roughness—all signs of aging that can be brought on by excessive sun exposure. It also works to clear up acne.

TRISH TIP: *Some irritation in the form of redness and flakiness is normal when tretinoin is first used. Follow the advice of your physician when beginning use.*

RETINOL. A close relation to tretinoin, retinol is the over-the-counter vitamin A derivative. It improves skin texture and clarity, and reduces pore size, fine lines, and sun damage. It is also very effective at increasing the skin's moisture content.

VITAMIN C. In addition to its antioxidant properties, vitamin C stimulates the fibroblasts to produce more collagen and elastin. Studies have shown that vitamin C is most effective in L-ascorbic acid form, so when shopping for skin products with vitamin C, look for that term on the ingredient label. Packaging is important too, as vitamin C can oxidize very quickly when exposed to air and light. Store it in a cool, dark place.

A LAST WORD: ANTIOXIDANTS

FOR VITAMIN A AND C TO BE MOST EFFECTIVE, THEY SHOULD BE USED AT DIFFERENT TIMES (A.M./P.M. OR ON ALTERNATING DAYS) SO THEY DON'T COUNTERACT EACH OTHER.

LUNCH TREATS

*Got an hour? Why not go to your dermatologist for an in-office treatment
that will make a difference with virtually no downtime.*

I. AHA PEEL
To diminish fine lines, even out pigmentation, and clear up acne, most people
undergo a series of six peels, each increasing the concentration and contact time
on the skin. Glycolic peels give you a smoother, brighter, and clearer complexion.
By sloughing off dead skin cells, they bring fresh new cells to the surface. For
maintenance, follow up once a month, or as your skin-care specialist recommends.

2. MICRODERMABRASION
This treatment, also known as a power peel, is helpful for improving skin texture,
unblocking pores, removing excess oil, and possibly reducing wrinkles and mild acne
scars. Sterilized aluminum oxide or sodium bicarbonate crystals are passed over
the skin, and, simultaneously, vacuum suction removes the particles along with debris
and dead skin cells. Better yet, you can apply makeup immediately after treatment.

3. FACIALS
There are many benefits to having regular facials: pores get professionally
cleansed, facial massage stimulates skin microcirculation, and, best of all, you feel
relaxed, which can only have a positive effect on how you look.

Have a facial in a dermatologist's office so that
any medical questions and concerns can be addressed
at the same time.

Why live with a pimple when a quick trip to the
dermatologist for a cortisone injection will clear it right up?

Invest in laser hair removal for your underarms, legs,
and bikini area. It will save you time in the future by
eliminating the need to shave or wax.

Have a full physical checkup for skin cancer.
Doing so can save your life.

SKIN-CARE QUICKIES

I

MAKE SURE YOU RINSE YOUR FACE THOROUGHLY
AFTER CLEANSING.

2

DO NOT OVEREXFOLIATE.

3

LEAVE YOUR BLEMISHES ALONE. REALLY, RESIST THE URGE
TO PICK. NO GOOD CAN COME FROM IT.

4

APPLY MOISTURIZER TO DAMP SKIN AND GIVE IT
A CHANCE TO ABSORB. DITTO FOR EYE CREAM.

5

DON'T RUB, ESPECIALLY AROUND THE EYES.

6

SLEEP, WATER, EXERCISE, A NUTRITIOUS DIET,
AND LIVING A BALANCED, HAPPY LIFE ARE THE BEST
BEAUTY TREATMENTS OF ALL.

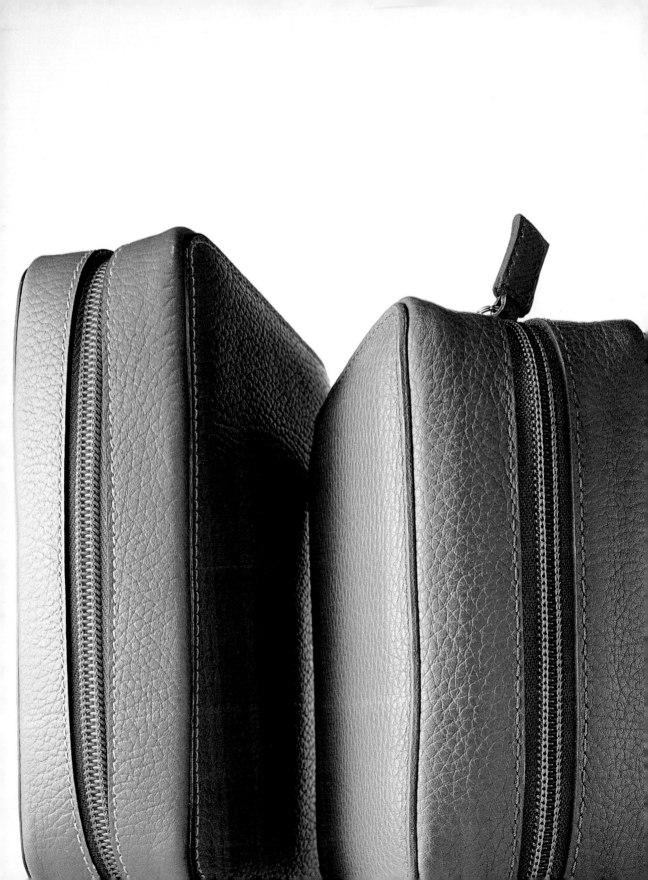

ORGANIZATION: *A Tale of Obsession*

A QUEST FOR ORDER

I ADMIRE ORGANIZATION IN OTHER PEOPLE. WHEN I MEET EXCEPTIONALLY ORGANIZED PEOPLE, I FIND MYSELF STUDYING WHAT THEY'RE DOING AND HOW THEY'RE DOING IT. I'M ALWAYS ON THE LOOKOUT FOR A NEW TIP THAT WILL MAKE LIFE EASIER, QUICKER, AND PRETTIER. (NEATNESS SIMPLY LOOKS BETTER.) SHIP-SHAPE PERSONALITIES NEVER LOOK FLUSTERED. THEY RARELY ASK FOR PENS OR PANIC AS THEY SHIFT THROUGH PAPERS. NOR DO THEY LEAVE ESSENTIAL ITEMS AT HOME. WE COULD SIMPLY ENVY THEM, BUT I FIND IT'S FAR MORE USEFUL TO LEARN FROM THEM.

I'm obsessed with order and placement because I'm a collector—shoes, clothes, books, you name it. I like to have a lot of choices around me, and I hold on to everything for the proverbial "just in case." Yet at the same time, I want to simplify and pare down. I want to make life easier, to have exactly what I need in front of me when I need it. For that, you need a system.

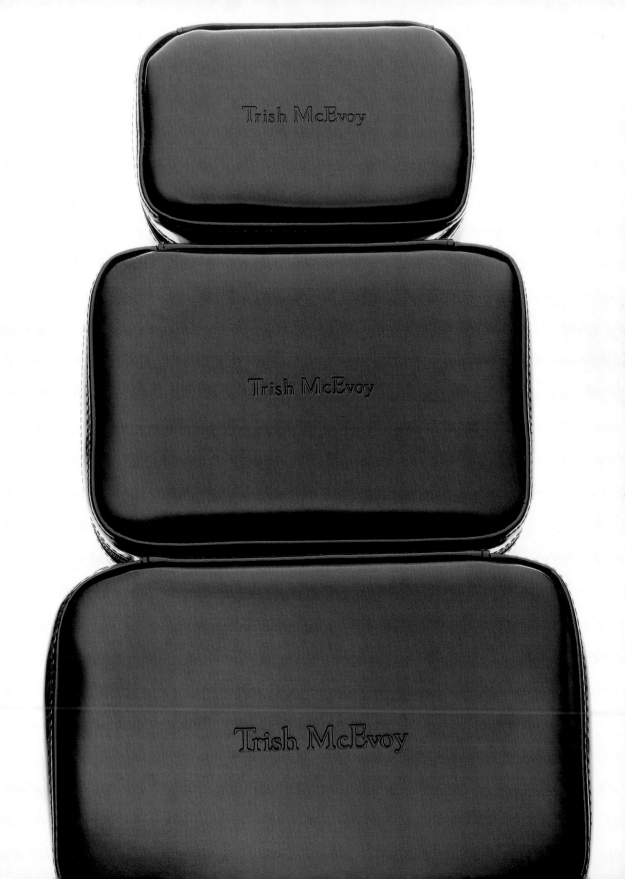

THE CREATIVE JOURNEY

MY FIRST SYSTEM WAS SIMPLY A ZIP-UP LEATHER BINDER WITH POCKETS SIZED FOR MY MAKEUP. BUT ALL THE DIFFERENT COMPACTS TOOK UP A LOT OF ROOM, AND I WAS CONSTANTLY OPENING AND CLOSING THEM, SEARCHING FOR JUST WHAT I WANTED. I SAT DOWN WITH MY TEAM—GERI EMMETT AND JOANNE PIGOZZI—AND THOUGHT ABOUT THE BINDER SOME MORE. WE INCLUDED "PAGES" THAT WOULD HOLD SQUARES OF MAKEUP SO THAT YOU COULD SEE ALL OF THEM AT ONCE WITHOUT HAVING TO TWIST OFF CAPS OR OPEN UP A TON OF COMPACTS. WE ALSO OFFERED AN OPTIONAL MESH BAG FOR PRODUCTS AND TOOLS THAT DIDN'T FIT ONTO FLAT PAGES, AND WE CREATED A MINI POUCH TO HOLD AND PROTECT BRUSHES. VOILA! THE PLANNER WAS AS SLEEK AS IT WAS FUNCTIONAL.

Later, we realized that the Planner's size was a factor. Women don't come in one size and neither do their handbags or the quantity of products they use. So we introduced three Planner sizes: large, medium, and petite. I own and use all three: a large at home, a medium always packed and ready for travel, and a petite one for my handbag.

Finally, we had to choose the color. Originally, black seemed like the most practical, essential color to offer. But many of us delight in color, and black doesn't always work geographically. (It can be so New York.) I myself craved color. We now offer a virtual rainbow of choices. On a pragmatic level, I find a colored Planner visually pops out of a dark bag. Again, no more searching around.

THE PLANNER: A PORTABLE, ALL-IN-ONE VANITY

I've found the Planner really helps me organize my makeup in the least amount of space possible. This is key, because most women I know hate being weighed down. You carry enough stuff around with you already; the Planner ensures that you carry just what you need. I edit what's in my Planner depending on where I'm going. If I'm heading to a warm-weather location, my makeup needs are very different than they are on a brisk day in New York City.

Another critical point about the Planner: you can organize the pages in the same order you put on your makeup. If concealing dark circles under your eyes is most important to you, that page comes first. Or if you're always touching up your lipstick, you may want to put the lipstick page on top. By organizing the Planner to suit your needs, you simplify your routine. The Planner is as much about customization as it is about form and function.

Has the Planner reached the end of its development? Probably not. For me, everything is a work in progress with room for improvement. I'm always raising the bar for myself. Yet because of the Planner's adaptability and flexibility, it's pretty near perfect. For now.

PLANNER - - - - - - - - - - - - - - - - - -

The all-in-one makeup organizer that holds makeup in one space-saving place. Convenient to use, the Planner keeps things clean, accessible, and tidy. The all-around zipper makes sure it all stays put.

LUCITE PAGE - - - - - - - - - - - - - - - -

These magnetic pages allow you to customize your own makeup look, and they give you at-a-glance visibility. They also give you the ability to change or refill colors as needed.

SIDE POCKET - - - - - - - - - - - - - - - -

This handy pocket with a Velcro closure enables you to store makeup accessories such as a puff, sponge, eyelash curler, or any other miscellaneous tool. It's also the perfect place to stash lipsticks.

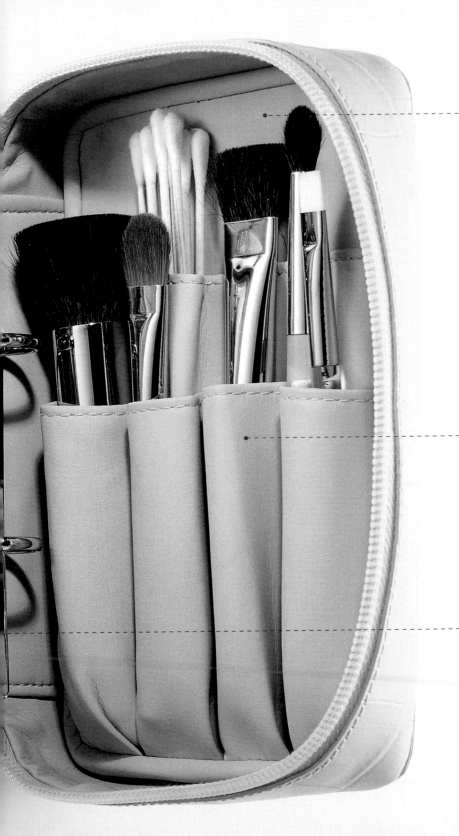

HIDDEN COMPARTMENT
This nifty back pocket holds larger or harder-to-hold items, such as compacts and mascaras as well as blotting papers and cotton swabs.

BRUSH SLEEVE
There is simply no better way to protect, store, and carry your brushes. The brush sleeves are sized to accommodate different thicknesses to ensure each brush is held securely.

BINDER RINGS
The Planner's backbone. Like any looseleaf binder, the rings securely hold the Lucite pages in place while allowing you the flexibility to add and remove pages as the seasons change.

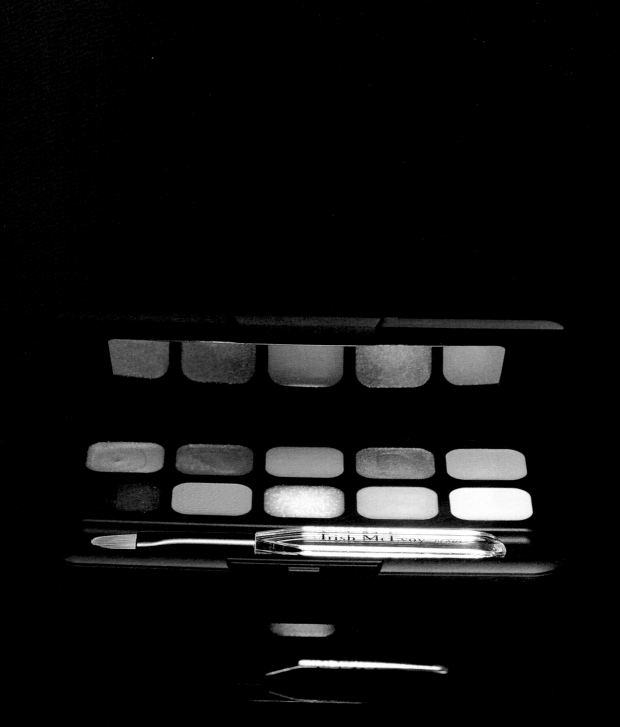

MAKEUP IN THE PALM OF YOUR HAND

THERE ARE SOME WOMEN WHO DON'T WANT TO CARRY EVEN AS MUCH
AS MY PETITE PLANNER. IT COULD BE THAT THEIR BAGS ARE TOO SMALL FOR
ANYTHING BIGGER THAN A COMPACT. PERHAPS THEY DON'T CARRY A BAG
AND ONLY HAVE A POCKET FOR PERSONAL POSSESSIONS.

My feeling is this: if you're limited to a compact, you should make the most of it. That's what led me to create my trademark specialty kits. These edited and refillable palettes of makeup are packaged in the sleekest, slimmest, credit card–sized compacts. They can be your main source of makeup or reserved for on-the-go touch-ups. I even have a compact with a double layer, so you can store even more makeup inside. Always look for products that speak to your lifestyle. The more user-friendly an item is, the more you will use it.

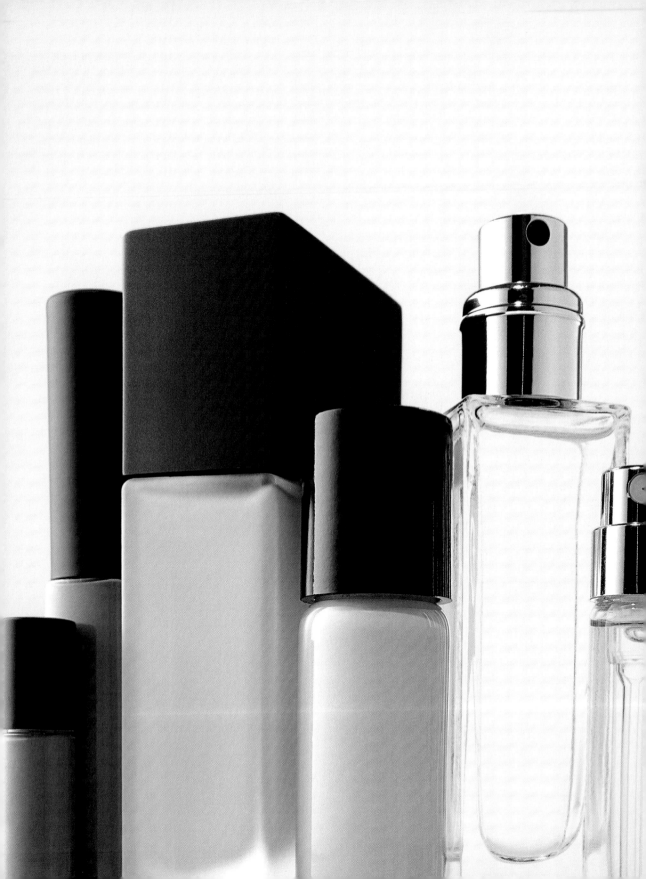

BEAUTY WHERE AND WHEN YOU NEED IT

IF YOU CAN, BUY DUPLICATES OF WHAT YOU LOVE MOST, BE IT A FOUNDATION, AN EYE PENCIL, OR A LIPSTICK. HERE'S WHY: IF YOU CAN LEAVE A PRODUCT PACKED IN A PARTICULAR LOCATION, IT WILL BE ONE LESS THING FOR YOU TO THINK ABOUT. FOR EXAMPLE, CREATE A MINI MAKEUP CASE TO LEAVE IN YOUR GYM LOCKER OR BAG. IF YOU LIVE OUT OF TWO HANDBAGS, BUY A LIPSTICK FOR EACH. IF YOU TRAVEL A LOT, AS I DO, KEEP A TRAVEL CASE PACKED AND READY TO GO. FOR THE PRICE OF AN EXTRA PRODUCT, YOU CAN SAVE LOTS OF TIME AND HAVE PEACE OF MIND EVERYWHERE YOU GO.

CLEAN UP, CLEAN OUT

HOWEVER YOU ARRANGE YOUR MAKEUP,
THE GOAL IS TO ORGANIZE YOURSELF SO THAT YOU CAN
CONCENTRATE ON APPLYING IT WELL.

You can't imagine what I help weed out of my clients' makeup bags, and they thank me every time. Ditch all those cosmetics you bought that weren't quite right. Toss anything that smells funny (cream formulas separate over time). Makeup has a shelf life of a year, with the exception of mascara, which should be replaced every three months, six at the most.

Check to see that your makeup is squeaky clean. Everything from brushes and sponges to powder puffs should be in pristine condition. Sharpen your eye and lip pencils. If you have a few lipsticks in rotation, slice off their tips now and then to uncover the fresh pigment.

My other editing rule is simple: if you don't love it, lose it. If you haven't worn it in six months, you're not likely to start now.

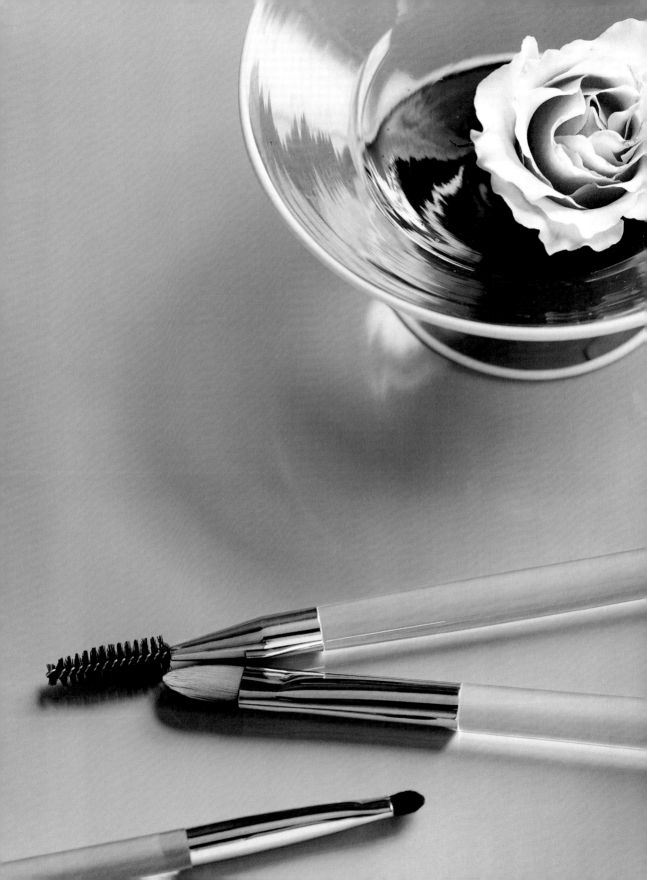

BRUSHES: *A Love Story*

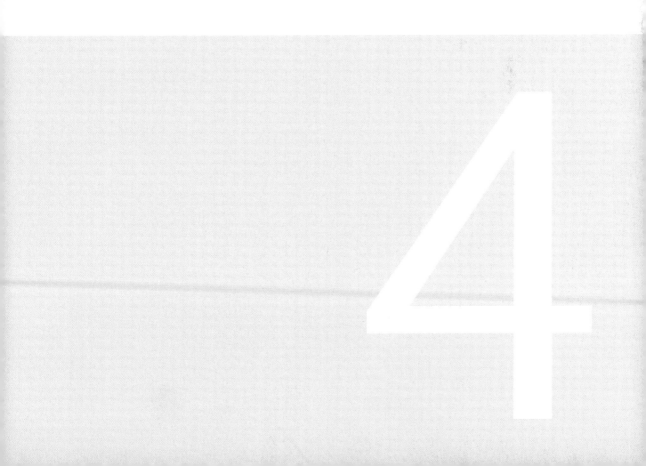

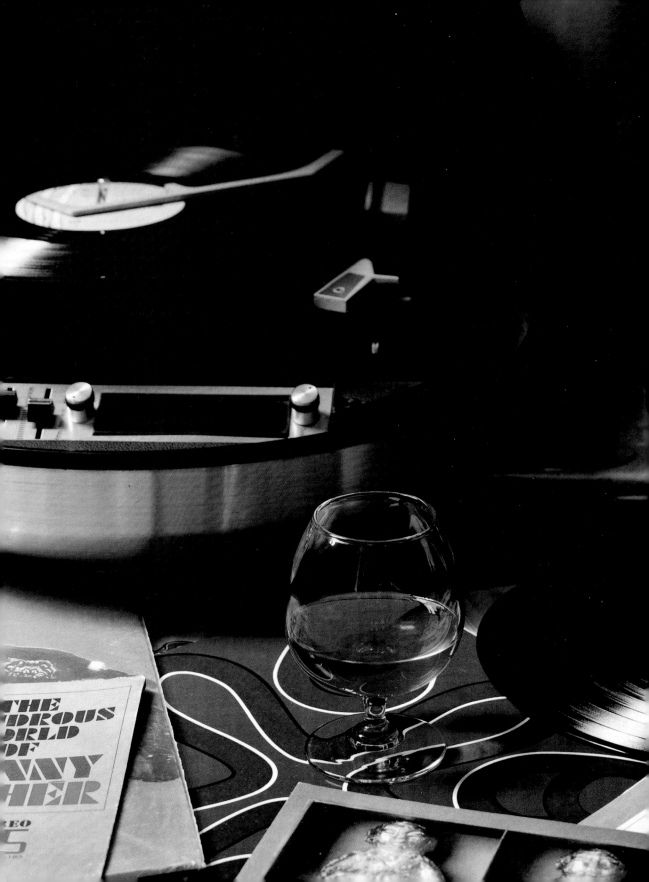

HARD TO BELIEVE, BUT MUSIC DIDN'T ALWAYS COME ON CDS. THERE WERE THINGS CALLED RECORDS, EIGHT-TRACKS, AND CASSETTE TAPES. MOVIES WEREN'T ALWAYS ON DVDS EITHER. YOU WATCHED VIDEOS OR, BEFORE THAT, FILM ON REELS. WELL, I'M HERE TO TELL YOU THAT MAKEUP BRUSHES WEREN'T ALWAYS THE NORM. WHEN I STARTED DOING MAKEUP, IT WAS DIFFICULT TO FIND GOOD TOOLS. COSMETIC COMPANIES DIDN'T SELL SEPARATE BRUSHES, ONLY THE ONES THAT CAME IN THE COMPACT. CREATING A BEAUTIFUL FACE WITH THOSE BRUSHES WAS A CHALLENGE, TO SAY THE LEAST. MAKEUP IS LIKE PAINTING: YOU'RE NOT GOING TO GET A PRECISE LINE UNLESS YOU HAVE THE PROPER INSTRUMENTS.

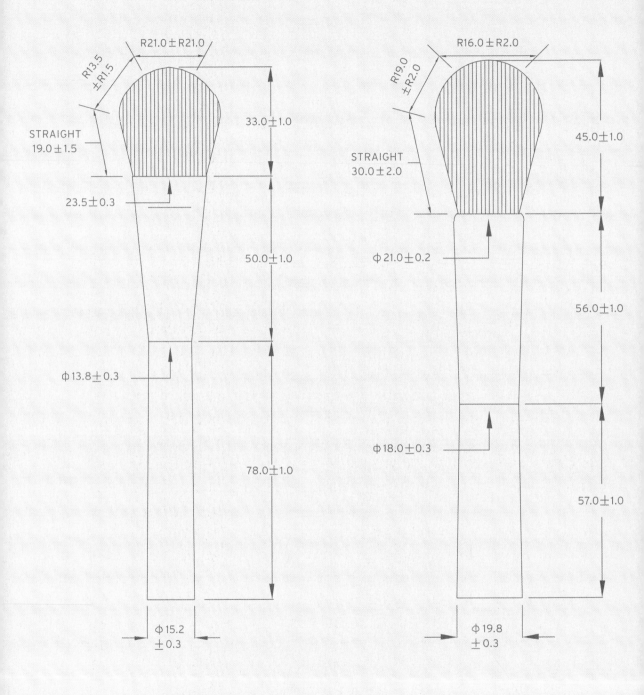

R21.0 ± R21.0

R13.5 ± R1.5

STRAIGHT 19.0 ± 1.5

33.0 ± 1.0

23.5 ± 0.3

50.0 ± 1.0

Φ13.8 ± 0.3

78.0 ± 1.0

Φ15.2 ± 0.3

R16.0 ± R2.0

R19.0 ± R2.0

STRAIGHT 30.0 ± 2.0

45.0 ± 1.0

Φ21.0 ± 0.2

56.0 ± 1.0

Φ18.0 ± 0.3

57.0 ± 1.0

Φ19.8 ± 0.3

CUSTOMER : TRISH MCEVOY	DESCRIPTION : 2B
DATE : 10 / JUN / 2003	MATERIAL
DRAWING NO : BSK30610-DWG837	-HAIR : SQUIRREL
SCALE : 1 : 1	-FERRULE : BRASS
UNIT : MM	-HANDLE : ACRYLIC

CUSTOMER : TRISH MCEVOY	DESCRIPTION : #37
DATE : 10 / JUN / 2003	MATERIAL
DRAWING NO : BSK30610-DWG838	-HAIR : SQUIRREL
SCALE : 1 : 1	-FERRULE : BRASS
UNIT : MM	-HANDLE : ACRYLIC

Off I went to the art store. I bought a handful of paintbrushes and began shaping them with a scissor. It was all trial and error. I realized if I cut the bristles shorter, it had one effect on application; if I left them longer it had another. The same was true if I cut them on an angle or to a very fine tip. Some of the wood handles were so long, I had to position my hand too far away from my body. So I broke them—problem solved. A new world opened up to me. Not only could I apply makeup better, I had fun doing it. These custom brushes felt good in my hand and even better on my skin. Most of all, I could truly control the makeup I put on my clients.

I look back and realize that those rudimentary brushes were the makeup equivalent of cranking the Victrola. But those brushes were to form the backbone of my business. I went to a manufacturer, and we started with six brushes: a blush brush, a powder brush, a base eye shadow brush, a crease brush, a concealer brush, and a lip brush. Over the years, I played with different hairs: sable, squirrel, pony, and then synthetics, which are great for creams and detail eyeliner work. I experimented with shapes and materials for handles. As I discovered new makeup needs, I added more brushes to the mix. Clients were clamoring for my brushes. So were other makeup artists. Not only did they love how the brushes felt against their skin, they also loved how easy they were to use and the professional results they created. Brushes are like sports equipment: the better the equipment, the better your game. Think of the difference between rented skis or bicycles and the ones that you own. It's all in the form and function.

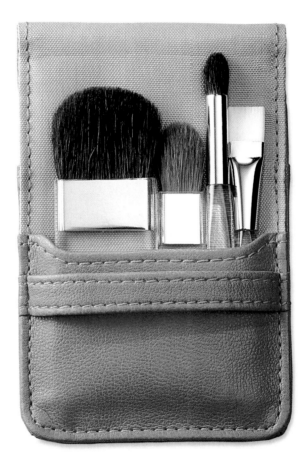

My love for brushes has never diminished. When you apply your makeup with a good brush, it feels wonderful, like the feeling you get from putting on a great cashmere sweater. You're an artist, and your face is your personal canvas. Applying makeup is a uniquely sensual experience, in which you really get to pamper yourself. A good brush is a precious, handmade instrument. Merely holding one makes you feel creative and glamorous.

Women are very particular about their makeup brushes. How they use them really comes down to personal style. Some women want their brush collection pared down to the core four or five essentials; others like owning an entire palette of them, delighting in the nuances of application. Let me assure you, there is no right or wrong. I can appreciate the need to own just a few favorites, and I also understand the desire to luxuriate in a full range of choices. I can also offer suggestions and guidelines.

BUY THE BEST YOU CAN AFFORD.
This is the place to splurge. The better the brush, the better the application.
Your makeup will speak for itself. With care, a good brush lasts a very long time.

TAKE YOUR HANDS INTO CONSIDERATION.
I have small hands, which is why I like short-handled brushes for doing my own
face. (When I do yours, I use longer handles because it's a vastly different experience.)
If you have a large palm, you're going to want something that fills it.

THINK ABOUT WHERE THE BRUSH WILL LIVE.
Are you buying it for your makeup vanity? Your purse? To travel with? Or will
you want the brush to go everywhere you do? There's a big difference between a
long-handled brush and a mini brush designed to fit into your makeup case.

DO YOU NEED IT TO APPLY MORE THAN ONE KIND OF MAKEUP?
Dual-purpose brushes are fine, but don't forget to clean them thoroughly with each use.

DO YOU LIKE HOW IT FEELS IN THE HAND AND AGAINST THE SKIN?
For me, this is the ultimate test. Brushes are tactile. If one is scratchy or brittle, move
on. If it feels clunky, you're not going to enjoy holding it.

ARE THE BRISTLES THE RIGHT LENGTH?
The shorter the bristles, the more makeup the brush will deposit on your skin.
Longer bristles will give you more of a wash of color.

ALWAYS GIVE IT A TAP.
After your brush touches the product but before it touches your skin, give it a tap or
remove excess product with a tissue. This way you start your application with exactly
the amount of color you need—no more, no less.

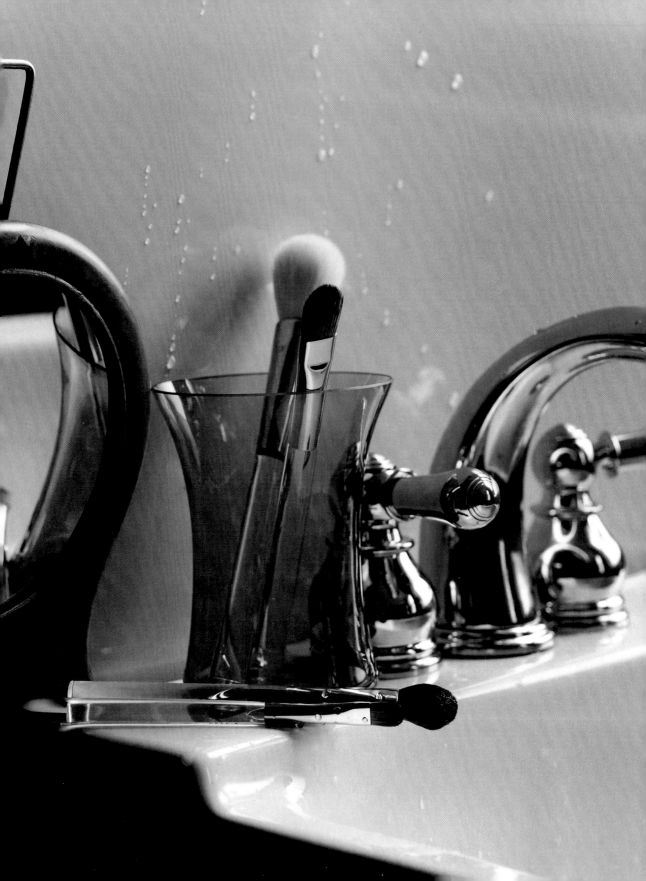

BRUSHES NEED TO BE WASHED REGULARLY.

Ideally, you should clean them from once a day to once a week. (I'm fanatical; I spray mine with brush cleaner after every use.) Use your own judgment and common sense as a guide. Look at and feel your brush. Is it matted with product buildup? If so, application will suffer. To wash, use a shampoo formulated for brushes. It will break down the makeup collected in the brush quickly and effectively. Put a little shampoo in your hand, then gently but thoroughly swish the brush in your palm. (Just don't get the metal barrel wet or bristles may begin to shed.) After washing, rinse thoroughly in clean water for a few moments and press out the excess moisture with a towel. Reshape as you would a wet sweater. Lay the brush flat on a sink, the head hanging over the edge so that air can reach the bristles. Trust me, it's worth the few minutes to clean a brush properly. You'll greatly extend its life and effectiveness.

EYE BRUSHES

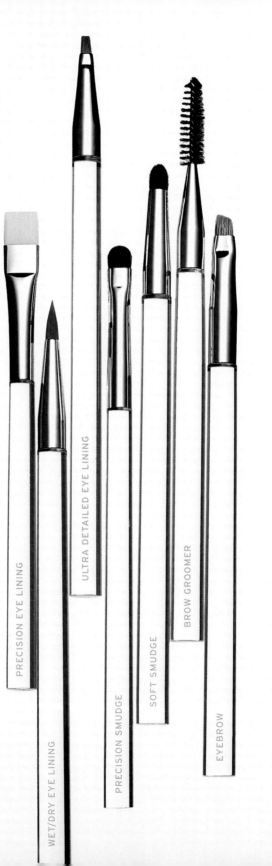

PRECISION EYE LINING

WET/DRY EYE LINING

ULTRA DETAILED EYE LINING

PRECISION SMUDGE

SOFT SMUDGE

BROW GROOMER

EYEBROW

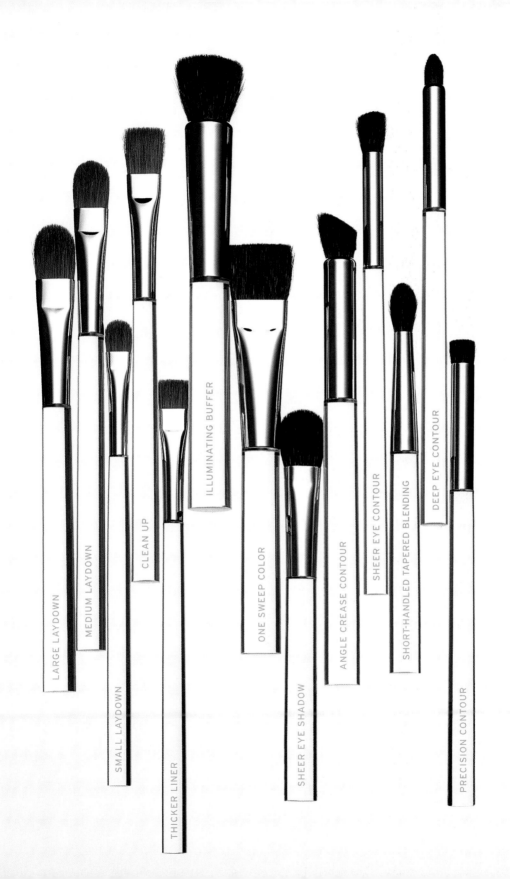

LARGE LAYDOWN

MEDIUM LAYDOWN

SMALL LAYDOWN

CLEAN UP

THICKER LINER

ILLUMINATING BUFFER

ONE SWEEP COLOR

SHEER EYE SHADOW

ANGLE CREASE CONTOUR

SHEER EYE CONTOUR

SHORT-HANDLED TAPERED BLENDING

DEEP EYE CONTOUR

PRECISION CONTOUR

FACE BRUSHES

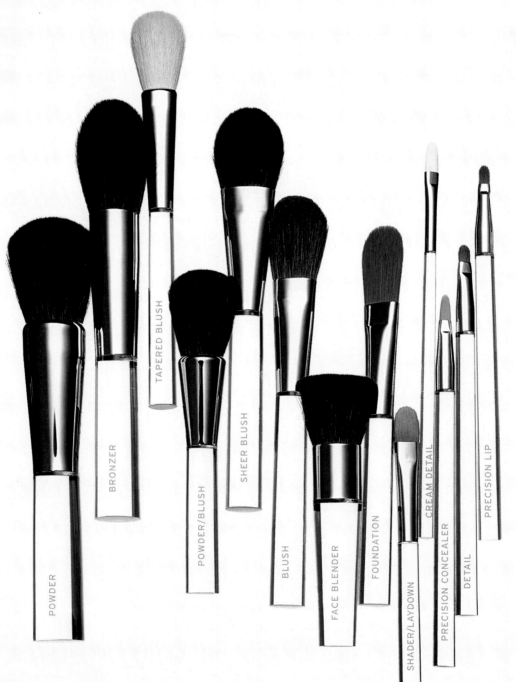

POWDER

BRONZER

TAPERED BLUSH

POWDER/BLUSH

SHEER BLUSH

BLUSH

FACE BLENDER

FOUNDATION

SHADER/LAYDOWN

CREAM DETAIL

PRECISION CONCEALER

DETAIL

PRECISION LIP

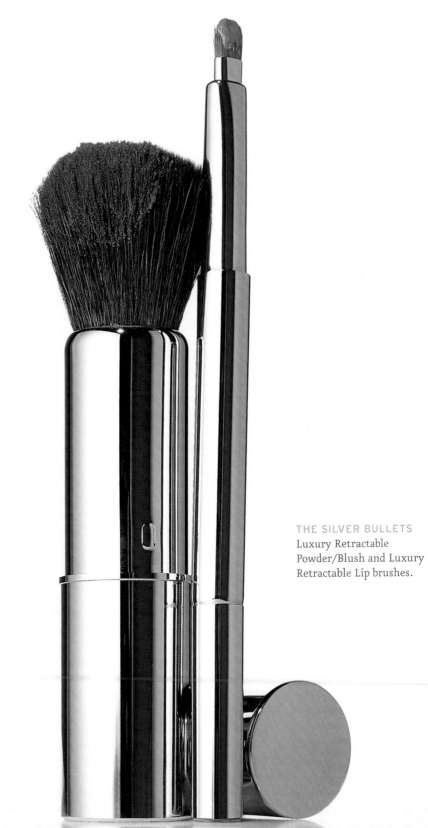

THE SILVER BULLETS
Luxury Retractable
Powder/Blush and Luxury
Retractable Lip brushes.

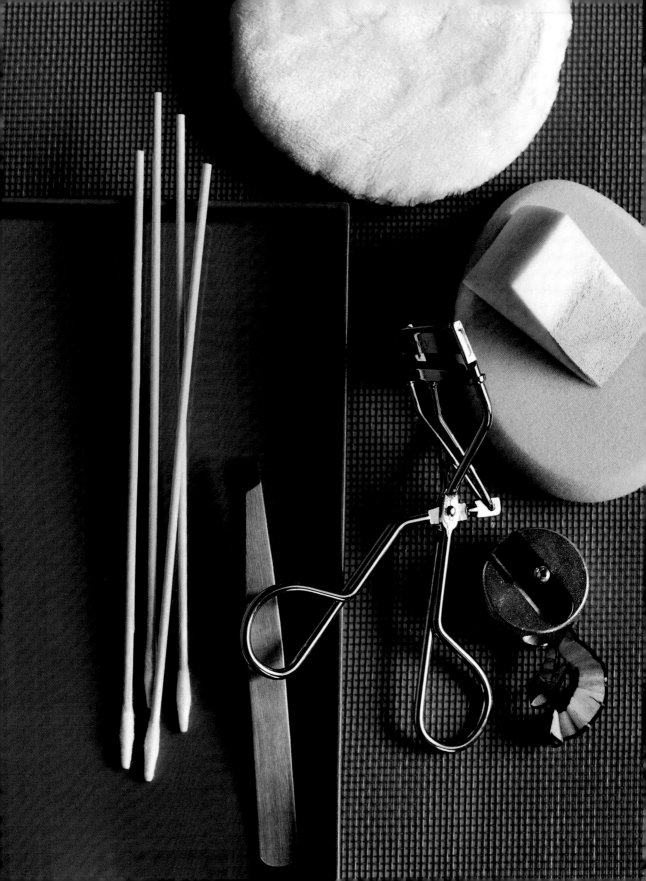

TOOLS THAT MATTER

AS IMPORTANT AS BRUSHES ARE, THERE ARE OTHER TOOLS YOU'LL FIND INVALUABLE. HERE ARE SOME OF MY ALL-TIME FAVORITE ESSENTIALS. THESE ARE ALL THE TOOLS YOU'LL EVER NEED TO APPLY MAKEUP BEAUTIFULLY.

COTTON SWABS
Look for tightly wound cotton with a rounded head (to remove makeup) or a slightly pointed tip (for detail work). I prefer the kind with longer wooden handles.

SPONGES AND WEDGES
Available either triangular or oval-shaped. Triangular-shaped are usually disposable and great for getting into tight corners when applying foundation, cream blush, and powder. Oval-shaped do all of the above and cover a lot of territory when applying or blending foundation, but they are not as good for getting into tight corners. The advantage of oval sponges is that they're long lasting and washable.

PUFF
Gives more coverage than a brush for powder application. Also, puffs help blend and remove any lines of demarcation. Look for one that's washable and made of velour.

EYELASH CURLER
Instantly gives a noticeable lift to the eyes' overall look. Pick ones that are curved and have rounded rubber pads.

TWEEZERS
I like the slanted kind because they give you a good grip.

PENCIL SHARPENER
Because what good is a pencil if it isn't sharpened?

MIRROR, MIRROR

The right mirror is among your more important tools. A bathroom mirror is fine, but in an ideal world, I'd love for you to have a mounted or a standing mirror that tilts and that has one side magnified (to whatever magnification you need). If that's not possible, a handheld magnifying mirror will work. Often, you need to zero in on what you're doing. This is true especially for eye makeup, where fine details matter. What's more, you want to be able to lift your chin and look down, eyelid flat—a position that's easier to attain with a tilted mirror. Why a magnifying mirror? If you can make your makeup look good close up in a magnifying mirror, it'll look even better from a distance.

Some makeup mirrors come with lights that mimic the lighting in different settings. Instead of one of these, I would opt for using natural daylight as your light source. Makeup that looks good in daylight will look good anywhere. If that's not an option, try to put your makeup on in a light that's similar to the light in which you'll be spending your time.

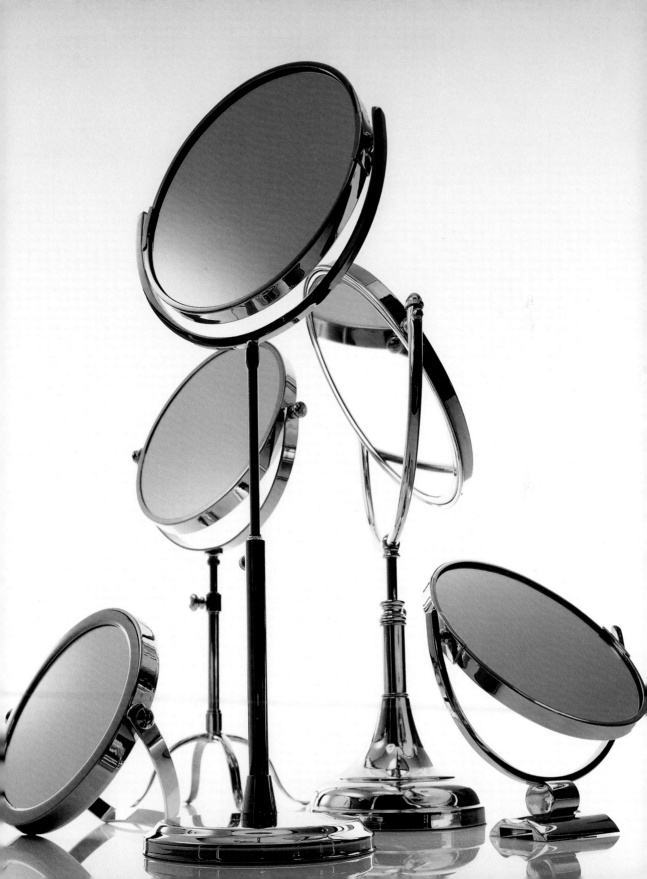

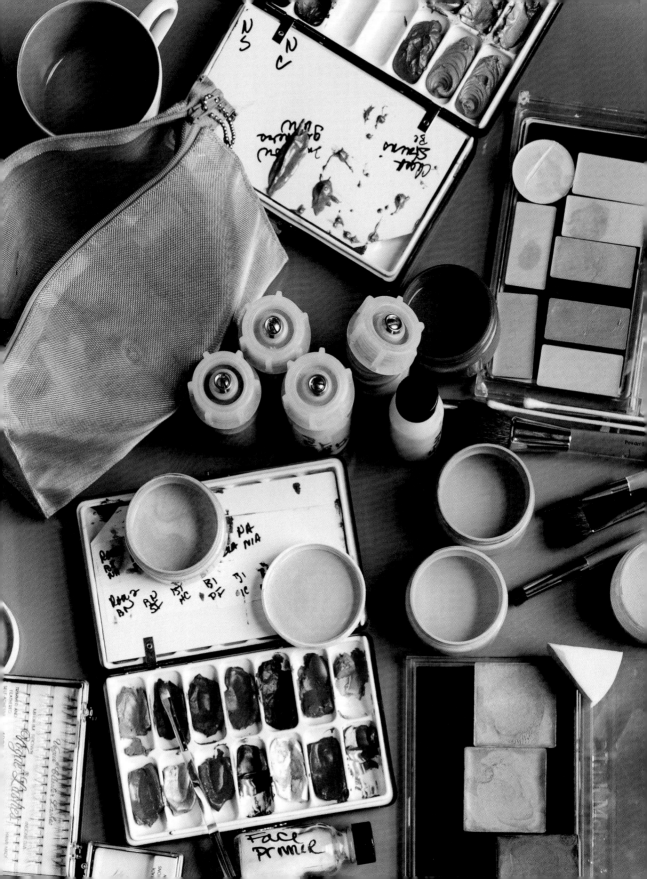

A GLOSSARY OF TEXTURES: *The Key to Look and Effect*

5

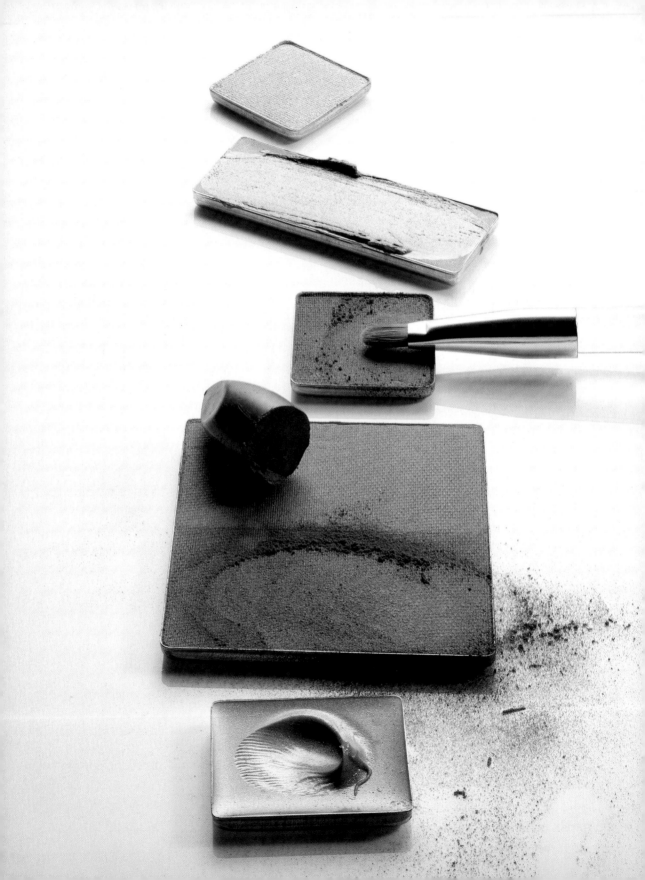

ONE OF THE THINGS I LOVE ABOUT OWNING MY OWN COSMETICS COMPANY IS BEING ABLE TO PLAY WITH COLORS AND FORMULAS TO COOK UP ANYTHING I CAN DREAM OF. MY ABSOLUTE FAVORITE THING IS TO EXPERIMENT WITH TEXTURE.

WHEN I DEVELOP A NEW PRODUCT, COLOR IS VERY IMPORTANT, BUT JUST AS IMPORTANT IS GETTING THE RIGHT TEXTURE. DO I WANT A SUEDE-LIKE OR A SILKY FEELING? DO I WANT THE PRODUCT TO APPEAR SHEER BECAUSE THE COLOR I HAVE IN MY MIND WILL HAVE A BETTER APPLICATION THAT WAY?

Think of your clothes. A white silk T-shirt is a whole different look than a white cotton T-shirt or a white cashmere T-shirt. A black wool dress says daytime, while a black sequined one screams evening. You wouldn't confuse the two while shopping. In comparing cosmetics, even though two colors look the same, they may look very different on, depending on their texture. Consider a sheer red lipstick versus a matte opaque one—two different looks, two different experiences.

Women will come to me and say, "I want a new eye look," but seldom do I hear "I'd like a semi-matte look" or "I really prefer shine in my makeup." I can make suggestions, but I'm better able to help you when I know what texture you're most comfortable wearing. The truth is that texture is the key to choosing a new eye look or a new lip style. If you don't have a knowledge of textures, you may feel lost when you're on your own at the makeup counter. You'll just keep experimenting away, hoping something "clicks," not knowing why a new product just doesn't seem to give you the effect you want.

My guess is that you probably have a grasp of the difference between warm and cool colors. (We'll talk more about color at the end of this chapter.) You also know what colors look good on you, and you have rightly made them part of your comfort zone. I want you to have that same appreciation of texture. It can make as big a difference as your color choices.

SKIN IS A TEXTURE

WHAT MAKES COSMETIC TEXTURE SO PIVOTAL IS THAT YOU COME INTO
MAKEUP WEARING A TEXTURE ALL YOUR OWN—YOUR SKIN. AS YOU KNOW,
THAT TEXTURE CHANGES DEPENDING ON THE DAY AND CLIMATE.
SOME DAYS YOU'RE DRY; OTHER DAYS YOU'RE NOT. WHAT YOU PUT ON YOUR
SKIN ON A GIVEN DAY IS GREATLY AFFECTED BY YOUR SKIN'S CURRENT
CONDITION AND THE CLIMATE YOU'RE IN.

For example, if your skin is feeling oily, you may reach for powder;
if it's dry, moisturized products will glide on better. Should you
find yourself in a warm, humid climate, even dry skin may find
that a powder blush has more staying power. Take the same skin
and put it in a dry, snowy climate, and I promise you a cream or gel
blush will simply work better. The more you understand your skin
and its needs, the easier it is to select a makeup texture.

TEXTURE IS A LOOK AND AN EFFECT

Thanks to technological advances in makeup, you have a wardrobe of textures to
choose from, whatever your skin type. A powder girl can find a powder that has a
velvety feel, so she gets the benefit of powder but the look she wants. A woman with
dry skin can wear a powder blush if she's properly prepped with a moisturizer.
Your texture choice is no longer solely determined by your skin type.

Texture has a striking effect on your makeup and can dress your look up
or down, just as it does with clothing. Once you know about textures, you are
empowered to make the right choices based on what works for you.

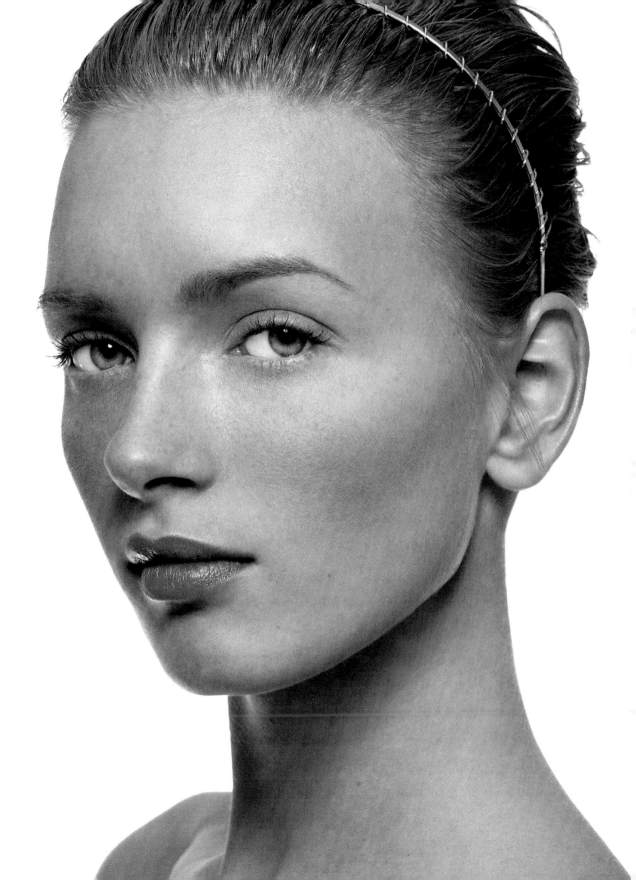

SHEER

Sheer products are the easiest to work with. You can't make
a mistake with sheer; there simply isn't enough pigment.
Sheer gives you the most natural effect because it allows skin to
show through. Sheer textures are not obvious; sometimes they
are barely detectable at all. Think of the words used to describe
sheer: a wash, a veil, a tint, a hint, a glow. All are more a
suggestion of color than an actual color. Sheer can be moist
to the touch, or sheer can be a powder.

SHEER TRUTHS

1. Sheer looks best when you dress casually.

2. Sheer is a great way to try a new color.

3. Sheer is the way to go when in doubt.

4. Sheer gives you a natural and relaxed look. It can give you a no-makeup look.

5. Sheer gives you less coverage.

6. Sheer doesn't last as long as matte. If you wear sheer, especially in lipstick,
you have to commit to more frequent touch-ups.

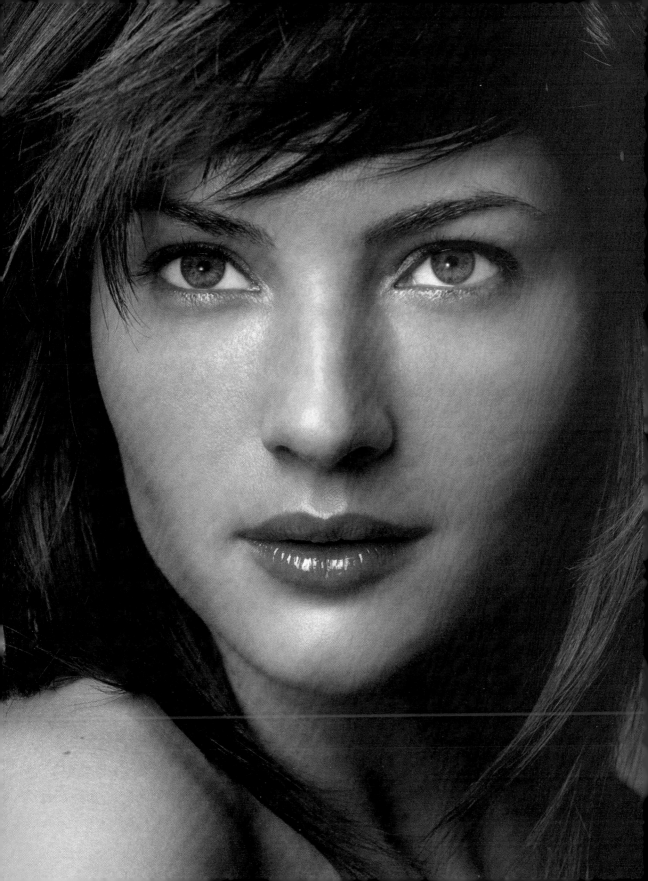

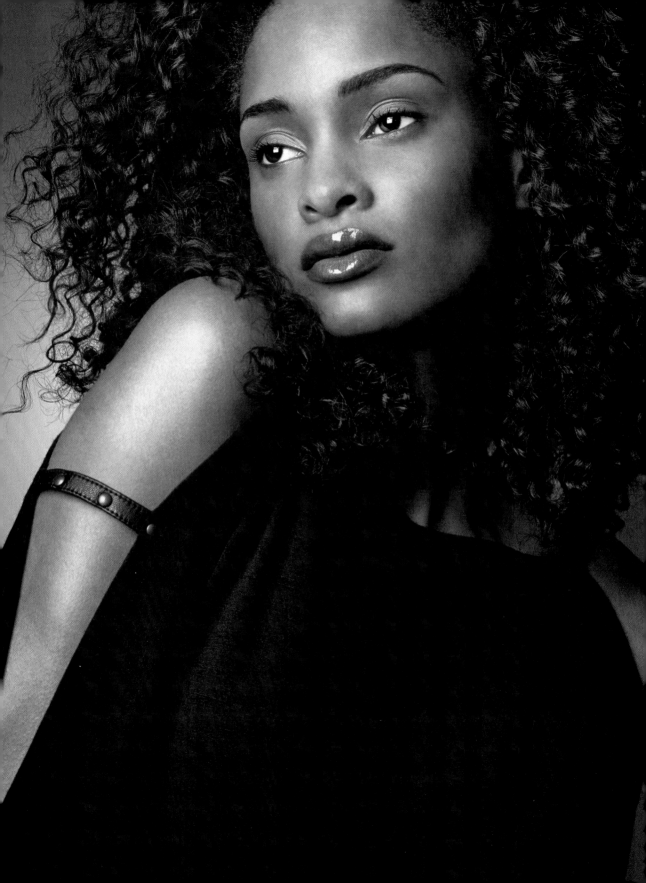

SHIMMER

Similar to sheer, a shimmer (sometimes called a luminizer) is a wash of subtle shine. Shimmers enhance whatever they touch and put radiance back into skin, what we call "the glow." Shimmers have light-reflecting properties, so they will draw attention to wherever they're worn. You want to put shimmer only on features you're feeling confident about and want to play up, such as eyebrow bones, cheekbones, and lips. Shimmers are so flattering, they look great on any age. They can work magic on older skin, adding the radiance and luminosity of younger skin.

When to avoid shimmers? Whenever you have something you'd rather not draw attention to, like fine lines, wrinkled eyelids, a blemish, a ruddy complexion, or any feature you'd rather downplay. Also, you want to add glow only where you don't shine naturally. Avoid the T-zone at all costs!

THE SHIMMER EFFECT

1. Shimmers highlight whatever they touch.

2. Shimmers can come in powder, cream, or liquid.

3. Shimmers enhance cheekbones.

4. Shimmer in a bronzer will give you a brighter, healthier glow.

5. Shimmer in a lipstick will create the illusion of fuller lips.

TRISH TIP: *A shimmer or luminizer gives the skin a translucent sheen. It can be applied with blush or mixed with foundation for a dewy, radiant finish. Again, apply a shimmer only where you aren't naturally shiny, such as on upper cheekbones and under the brow bones.*

MATTE

Matte is the absence of glow. In makeup terms,
matte usually translates into denser coverage and a drier finish.
The opposite of shimmer, matte buffs whatever surface it's
applied to. For example, if you're prone to a shiny forehead, you'd
be wise to reach for a matte powder. Not surprisingly, eyeliner
powders tend to be matte, and one of the dressiest lipsticks you
can wear is a semi-matte. Older women should use matte texture
strategically, where they need makeup with longevity, and in
combination with sheer and shimmer.

MATTE MATTERS

1. Matte gives the most coverage.

2. Matte is denser and therefore more dramatic.

3. Matte is longer lasting.

4. Matte feels and looks drier on skin, which makes it ideal for oily complexions.

5. Matte deflects attention.

TRISH TIP: *Matte has its clear advantages.*
So many clients had told me that their eyeliner smudged and didn't last very long—
a real problem if you depend on your liner.

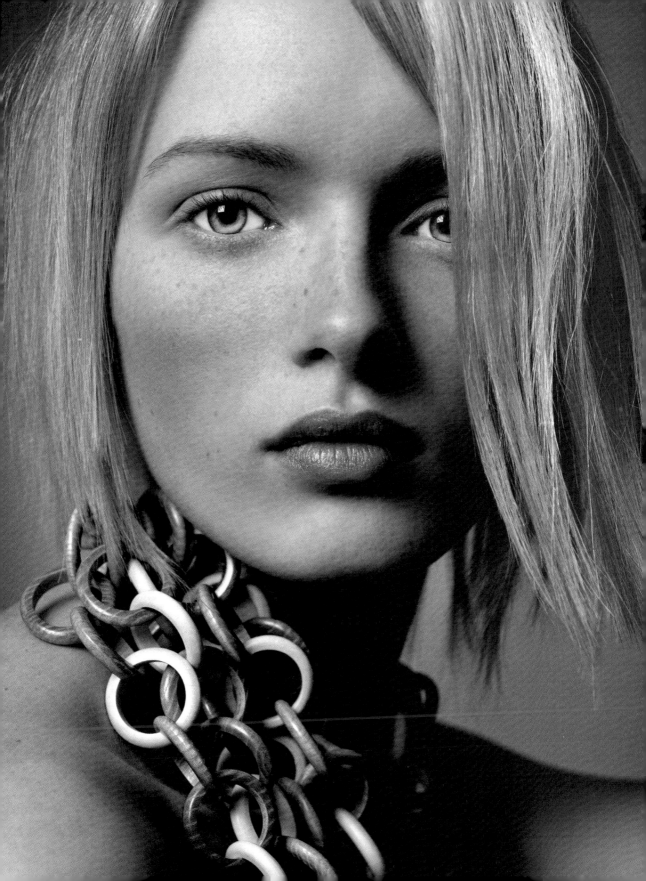

COVERAGE

COVERAGE BEGINS AND ENDS WITH TEXTURE. WHEN SELECTING FOUNDATION, CONCEALER, OR POWDER, YOU MUST FIRST ASK YOURSELF HOW MUCH COVERAGE YOU NEED. SOMETIMES YOU JUST WANT TO NEUTRALIZE OR TONE DOWN CERTAIN AREAS OF THE SKIN; OTHER TIMES YOU WANT TO ELIMINATE EVEN THE SUGGESTION OF A RED BUMP OR DARK SPOT. MOST TIMES, HOWEVER, YOU SIMPLY WANT TO EVEN OUT SKIN TONE. I SUGGEST YOU GO FOR THE COVERAGE YOU REQUIRE WHERE YOU NEED IT. IN A PINCH, YOU CAN OPT FOR "BUILDABLE" COVERAGE—ADDING MORE LAYERS OF A SHEER PRODUCT TO REACH A MORE OPAQUE COVERAGE. REMEMBER, SHEER IS MORE NATURAL; MATTE IS DENSER.

FOUNDATION

Tinted moisturizer. Ideal for a healthy glow and a hint of coverage. Best for clear skin because it won't cover uneven pigmentation. I developed a tinted moisturizer with an SPF 15 as an all-in-one product.

Cream-to-powder, water-based liquid formulas, or dual finish (wet/dry) are great for everyday application. Each allows for buildable coverage. The choice is yours.

TRISH TIP: *Foundation should never alter or add color to your skin. That's what blush and bronzers are for. Foundation's purpose is to even out and enhance your natural skin tone.*

CONCEALER

Nothing refreshes your look like concealer. Concealers take away shadows, make dark circles disappear, and diminish spider veins around the nose. I developed Even Skin concealer in two shades and textures. (The two colors are for custom blending to match variations in your skin tone.)

Creamy. Great for someone who needs more coverage than foundation offers alone and doesn't have a lot of fine lines.

Opaque. Most complete coverage and longest lasting; perfect for stubborn undereye darkness and blemishes.

TRISH TIP: *I'm often asked which comes first, concealer or foundation. Foundation comes before concealer. Always apply concealer in light layers and build coverage. Finish with a light dusting of powder.*

POWDER

For me, powder is simply a way of life. I use it for everything from blending makeup to setting makeup for longevity. Powder can be a big eraser of mistakes or the perfect finish.

Powder comes either loose or pressed. Loose powder is lighter and therefore gives you a sheerer application. It also contains no binders, which makes it especially good for problem skin. I have come to treasure my loose powder compact because it's convenient to carry around for touch-ups. I consider loose powder essential to any and all makeup. If your goal is primarily to set your makeup, go for a translucent, colorless powder.

Pressed powder offers the convenience of coming in a compact. Many times powder can stand in for foundation, especially when pressed on with a sponge.

Some women worry that powder will dry out their skin. Thanks to advances in technology, that's not a problem. Other women are worried that they will look powdery. Also not true. Powder can be buffed away to an invisible layer. Powder's texture has much to do with its application. I suggest sponges and puffs for more coverage, and a soft, long-haired powder brush for sheer coverage.

TRISH TIP: *Once a powder is applied, only other powder textures should be layered on top of it.*

BLUSH/BRONZER

Powder. Probably the most popular due to its ease of application. Great for all skin types, assuming skin is properly prepped. For best results, apply bronzer or blush over foundation and powder.

Cream. Very easy to work with and can be worn on bare skin. To apply, use fingertips, sponge, or brush.

Gel. Gives a transparent, natural glow. Needs to be applied to bare skin or over foundation. Don't use over powder.

Liquid. Longest wearing. Should be applied to bare skin. Because it's a stain, it requires practice to make perfect.

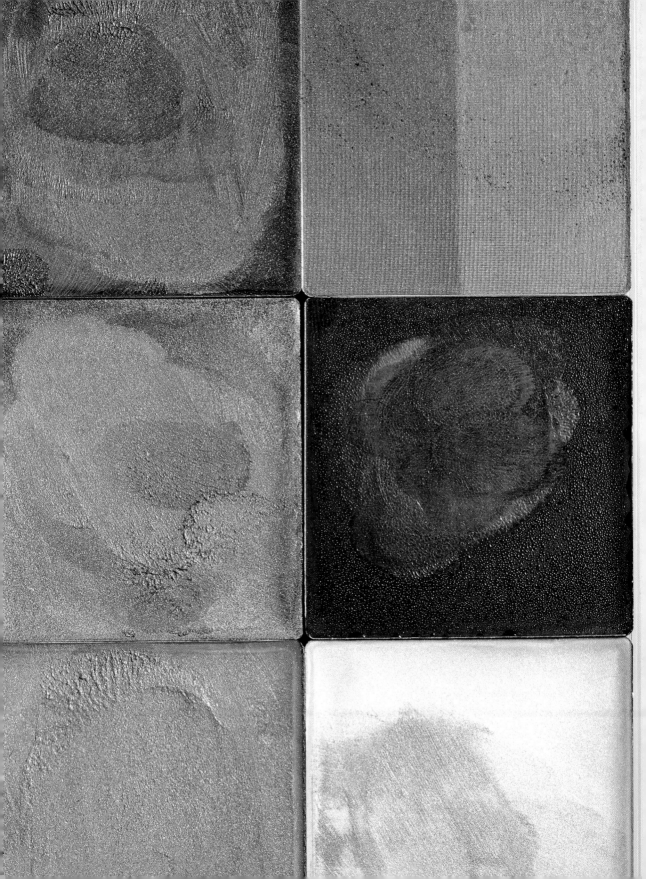

LIPS

WHEN IT COMES TO LIP COLOR, THE TEXTURE YOU CHOOSE IS AS IMPORTANT
AS THE SHADE. WITH LIPS, TEXTURE TRULY TELLS THE STORY.

GLOSS. Comes in many textures and colors, from sheer to opaque. Worn alone or over lipstick.

LIP BALM. When colorless, it's the perfect prep for lips. Now balms come in color, made to be worn on their own, and leave lips feeling smoother.

SHEER LIPSTICK. A wash of color, a sheer is somewhere between a gloss and a cream lipstick. Sheer is a great way to experiment with bold colors.

SUEDE LIPSTICK. Gives the same effect as a sheer but without the shine.

LIP STAIN. Transparent color, provides the longest wear. Lips should be prepped with lip balm before application.

CREAM LIPSTICK. The classic. Contains more pigment than a gloss or sheer, which makes it last longer.

SHIMMER LIPSTICK. One of the most popular. Great for giving lips a fuller look. Easy to apply. Also very forgiving.

SEMI-MATTE LIPSTICK. Has longer wearability than a cream, but is not as dry as a matte formula.

MATTE LIPSTICK. Has a no-shine finish.

LIP PENCIL. Used to define the lip. Can also be worn filled in on the lips for longer wear.

CHUBBY PENCIL. Available in all the various lipstick textures. Benefits of both lining and lip color.

EYE SHADOWS
YOUR CHOICE SHOULD BE INFLUENCED BY EFFECT AND WEARABILTY.

POWDER. The most popular. Comes in matte or glazed textures.

CREAM. Easy to apply because it needs less precision. Thanks to new technology, creams now wear longer than they used to. Can be applied with fingertips and brushes. Come in sticks, pans, and wands. Some formulas, like my Waterstix, are waterproof and come in matte or glaze textures.

GLOSS. Gives a shiny look to the eye. Great for photography, but in reality doesn't wear well and can look a bit messy.

CHOOSING COLOR

Color is grouped into two categories: warm and cool. Warm tones are those consistent with sunshine, such as yellow, orange, and peach, but the spectrum continues into neutrals like brown. Cool tones have the blue undertone of a cold day—white, mauve, lilac, blue, and eggplant.

While there may be no right or wrong color choices, some colors will flatter your particular skin tone more than others. There are a few guidelines that can help steer you to those color families. This isn't to say that you can't wear other colors or mix the color groups. But colors truest to your color family will better enhance your skin tone.

How do you know which color family is for you? Hold up the "warm" page under your chin and look into a mirror. Repeat the step with the "cool" page. One of these pages will instantly complement your skin more than the other. If you are unsure which color family is better for you, ask a friend to look at them with you.

WARM

COLOR CODING

1. A DARK SHADE MAKES SOMETHING RECEDE; A LIGHT ONE MAKES IT COME FORWARD.

One of the things you need to know when applying color is the power of light and dark. Dark adds depth and intensity; light adds softness and glow, just like a black dress will make you look sophisticated and thin, and a white one will make you look fresh and light you up. Darkness frames; lightness accentuates. With makeup, you need both. It's through the interaction of light and dark that you create a desired effect.

2. COLORS HAVE PERSONALITIES, EVEN SEASONS.

The intensity of a shade determines its impact. Dreamy, paled-down tones have an ethereal effect. Dark, kohl-rimmed eyes hint at seduction. The tropical punch of a vivid coral lipstick says summer like nothing else. Come winter, you may find yourself reaching for deeper tones, yet in the spring, a cheery peach or pretty pink feels more appropriate. Wear a pink lipstick on a gray day, and your whole look and mood will instantly lift. Color has power. Use it to your advantage.

3. NEUTRALS ALWAYS WORK.

You can't go wrong with a neutral. When in doubt, reach for shades of taupe, honey, plum, beige, or brown. They go with every coloring and every color.

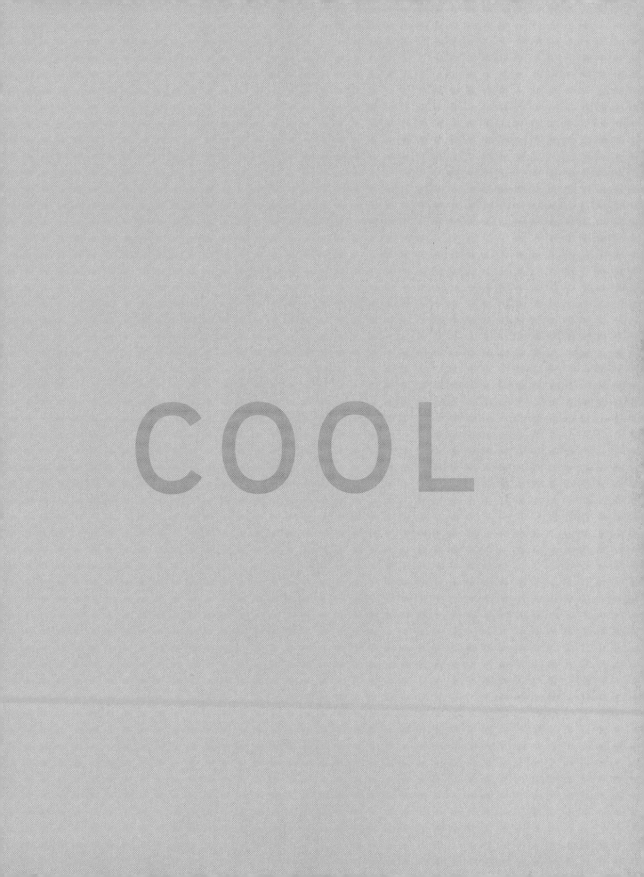
COOL

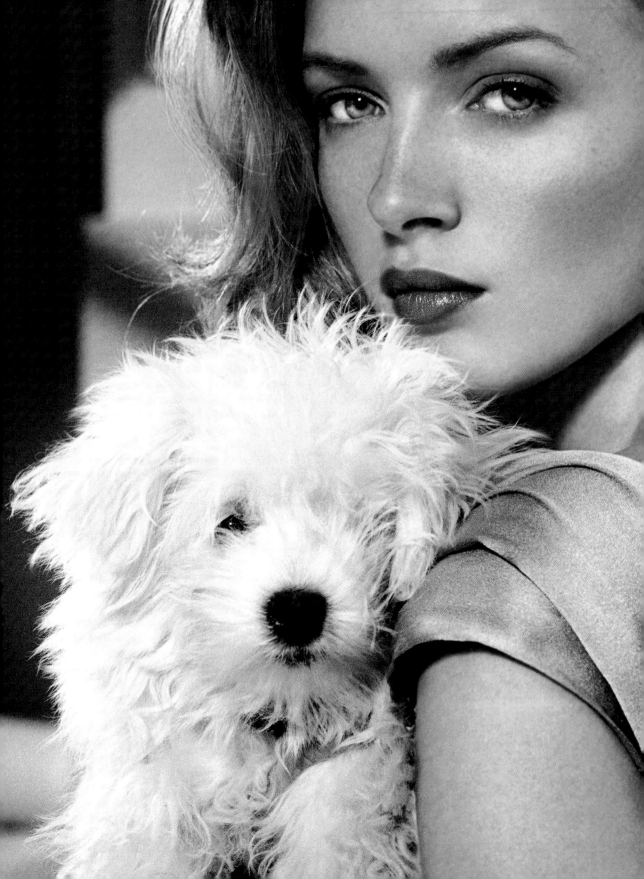

THREE LEVELS OF BEAUTY: *Application and Technique*

6

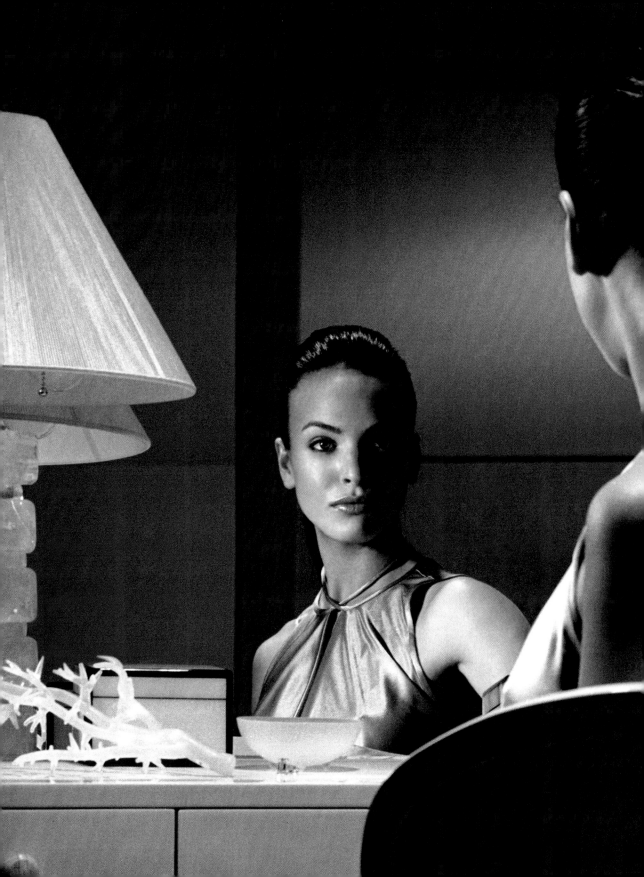

DETERMINING YOUR LEVEL

IF YOU COME TO ME FOR A CONSULTATION, I WILL ASK YOU QUESTIONS ABOUT YOUR LIFESTYLE. HOW MUCH TIME DO YOU REALLY HAVE FOR MAKEUP? DO YOU TRAVEL? WHAT KIND OF CLIMATE DO YOU LIVE IN?

THE MORE I KNOW ABOUT YOU, THE MORE I CAN HELP. IT'S HOW YOU SEE YOURSELF AND HOW YOU LIVE THAT MATTERS MOST. ONCE WE HAVE YOUR PRIORITIES DOWN, WE CAN GO TO WORK. I CAN CUSTOMIZE YOUR REGIMEN, AS WELL AS GIVE YOU A WARDROBE OF OPTIONS. IN MAKEUP, ONE SIZE DOES NOT FIT ALL. ONE SIZE DOESN'T EVEN FIT ONE PERSON. WE HAVE TOO MANY MOODS AND EXPRESSIONS. MAKEUP EVOLVES WITH YOU.

You may be thinking, of course I know my style. It's easy, however, to get stuck—that is, to think of yourself one way, maybe a way you were years ago, and not really take into account how you live now. For example, you may have been a Wall Street whiz, yet have recently taken time off to be an at-home mother. Those two roles require vastly different makeup approaches. I met a woman, Brita, who liked a fresh-faced look until she reached her forties. Suddenly, the natural look didn't work anymore. She needed to restore the definition that time takes away. Life is always changing, and so must your look.

My job as a makeup artist is to teach you about makeup that works for your life. If you live in very casual clothing, you probably like a minimally made-up face (Level One). If your style is little dressier, most likely you desire a more defined look (Level Two). And if you love to experiment with all kinds of looks and fashion trends, you're going to want to see your style through with your makeup (Level Three). This isn't to say that you won't wear khakis one day and a ball gown the next. But most of us have a signature style that we wear at least 80 percent of the time and feel most comfortable in. That's the look you want to address. That look is your Level.

Your Level determines which makeup and application techniques you choose.

AN HONEST ASSESSMENT

BELIEVE ME, THIS IS TRICKIER THAN IT SOUNDS AND YET SO VERY IMPORTANT. YOU'VE LIVED WITH YOUR FACE FOR A LONG TIME, STARED AT IT FOR HOURS IN THE MIRROR. YOU ASSUME IT CAN'T HOLD ANY SURPRISES. WRONG! WHAT YOU NEED IS DISTANCE AND OBJECTIVITY. THE MIRROR GIVES YOU ONE PERSPECTIVE, USUALLY A STATIC ONE (UNLESS YOU'RE THE TYPE WHO TALKS AND LAUGHS INTO IT).

Try looking at candid photos, ones in which you were caught off guard. Preferably, they should be photos from days on which you spent a lot of time and effort getting ready, maybe a holiday get-together or an office party. Photos capture both the big picture and the small details that the naked eye might miss. Even better, look at a videotape, where you can see yourself from all 360 degrees. Whatever you're looking at, you want to study it carefully to see what you can learn.

Let me tell you about such a photo. A few years ago I appeared in an ad campaign for Anne Klein called "Significant Women." Just the title and the women with whom I appeared made me feel great. But as fun as the experience was, I didn't love the resulting photo. There it was, in every magazine for all the world to see. Worse, I was blown up to billboard proportions. I loomed over New York City's Times Square. Talk about humbling moments! People said I looked good, but I knew I could look better. Off to work I went. I started with my hair, ditching the short haircut. I worked with my lab to develop an extra-coverage concealer, and I made an appointment with my husband for Botox. I used this experience to make changes I otherwise wouldn't have made.

The power to fine-tune your look comes from knowledge and objectivity. You need to be critical and detached, the way we all are when we study movie star photos in magazines. Ever notice how easy it is to assess someone else's face?

With a kind eye, look at a photo of yourself as you would one of a stranger. You'd probably notice first and foremost her general look, the impression she gives. Is this a woman comfortable in her skin? Is she smiling? Is she soft-looking? Are her features well defined? What about the color of her face? Could it be warmed up? Does her face tone match her neck? Be constructive, not critical.

The better you know yourself, your style, and what you want to enhance, the closer you are to realizing your Level best beauty.

You're a minimalist. Makeup is not a driving passion in your life. You want to throw it on and go. You want a bare-bones regimen, and you want to know only about products and techniques that are important to you. The most you want is one product per feature, two tops. Something to even out your skin tone, something to address an area that is bothering you or that you want to enhance. Maybe you'd like to cover blemishes and dark circles. Or wear mascara to bring out your eyes. Perhaps a new lipstick or gloss. Much more than that, and I lose you. You're simply not interested in having makeup be a huge part of your life. Yet the makeup you do wear is essential to you. It makes you feel dressed, it makes you feel finished. That's why you care enough to be reading this book or coming to my counter. I know you because I've always dreamed about being as carefree as you are about makeup. I applaud you for knowing who you are.

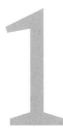

1

YOUR MAKEUP GOALS

To improve on nature. To even out skin tone.
To address areas that are bothering you.
To subtly dress up your face.

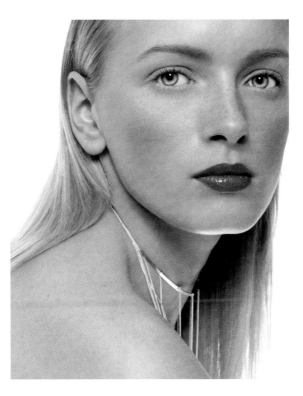

You enjoy makeup, and, what's more, you rely on it. In fact, you won't leave the house without it. Makeup's an essential part of your routine, like styling your hair. While Level One likes it simple, you kick it up a notch. You use makeup to enhance and define your look, as well as punch up your overall color. You wear at least two products per feature and are open to learning new techniques. You have an appreciation of how to work light and dark, and you like to switch around among a few lipstick colors. You don't want to look made up—you just want to look good. You have things you want to highlight and things you want to cover. I know you well because I'm a Level Two. I find most women fall into this category. We can also be a One or a Three, depending on the situation, but mostly we're comfortable somewhere in between.

2

To achieve a more defined look.
To highlight, cover, and enhance.

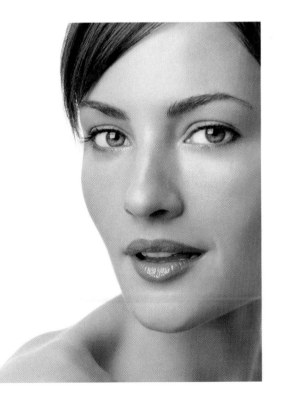

You love what makeup in all its extremes can do for you. With you, makeup is a creative journey, a means of expression. You like to play and have fun with it, slipping on one personality one day, another the next. You're not afraid to push the envelope to try a new look. You love the impact you get from high definition. You're more than happy to spend time on the details that make a difference. You appreciate the various effects different brushes give you, and you always take that extra step to achieve the precise look you're after. To you, the payoff is well worth it. You embrace the power of makeup in all its glory.

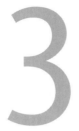

3

To maximize your beauty potential
through the artistry of makeup.

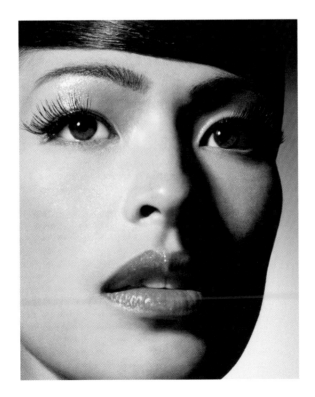

KEEP
IN MIND

I

LEVELS BUILD ON ONE ANOTHER.

Think of Levels as progressive steps. You have to graduate from one before moving on to the next. For example, you must master the fundamentals of Level One before you can move on to Level Two. And Level Three is the equivalent of makeup graduate school.

2

LEVELS ARE AGELESS.

Levels are really a question of time, lifestyle, and interest. I've met fourteen-year-old Level Threes and ninety-year-old Level Ones.

3

LEVELS ARE FLUID, ONE OFTEN MERGING INTO ANOTHER.

A Level One may become a Level Two for a special occasion. A Level Two may fall back to Level One on a more casual day, or bump up to Level Three for evening. But a Level One would probably not advance to a Level Three overnight, nor would a Three suddenly become a Level One.

4

YOUR LEVEL CAN CHANGE.

Levels don't typecast you for life. Levels are about lifestyles and how you want to look. You may gain more confidence with makeup and turn from a One into a Two. Sometimes Level Threes find themselves short on time and shed layers until they become more of a Level Two. Life's too short to limit yourself to one style forever.

You've identified your Level, your skin is prepped, and your makeup selected. Now you're ready to apply it. As discussed, you must master the Levels chronologically. You can't graduate from one Level, until you've mastered the one before it. Therefore, I'm going to walk you through makeup application Level by Level. Feel free to stop at your Level or pick and choose as you go along. Levels overlap. For example, a Level One may find herself trying on a Level Two eye application at night. Your Level is defined by your general approach to makeup; it's not an absolute.

BEFORE WE BEGIN. . .

Across-the-Level Guidelines for an Easier Application Process

Have all your tools in front of you. I developed the Planner to have easy access to my own makeup and to eliminate clutter. However you do it, don't wait until your application is under way to go hunting for brushes, sponges, or cotton swabs. It's helpful to have eye makeup remover within reach too.

Before applying makeup, prep your face with eye cream, moisturizer, and lip balm, and give your skin time to absorb them. You'll find they really set the stage. (I created a luxe lip balm with an SPF 15 that is wonderfully multifunctional because it provides moisture with sun protection, and it can be used on the lips or on the face.) Very important: Be sure to blot away any excess preparation product with a tissue.

Even if you put your makeup on in front of the bathroom mirror, have a handheld magnifying mirror nearby, especially for eye makeup, which needs attention to detail. In fact, you'd be wise to put on all your makeup using such a mirror. If your makeup looks good magnified, it'll only look better from a distance.

If you use your fingertips—and there are lots of times when it's the fastest, easiest method—be gentle! The goal is to tap and press, not to push and rub. Also, whenever only one finger is needed, use your ring finger. Since it's your weakest finger, it will help ensure that you press lightly. Otherwise, use a brush; brushes are great for details.

Blend, blend, blend. When it comes to any kind of face makeup—concealer, foundation, blush, bronzer—you must blend away all telltale edges. Not blending well is one of the most common mistakes I see. Depending on the product's texture, you can use a wet sponge or a big puff to help soften the effect. (Look for a puff made of the softest velour you can find, and make sure it's washable.) I will be telling you to blend and powder throughout this application section. It's that important!

I like to start most applications with the eyes. Why? Because as you put on eye makeup, product sometimes drops onto the face. It's far easier to clean up before you've put on concealer, foundation, and powder.

For eye application, you want to lift your chin and look down into the mirror. Try to keep your eye open. The goal is to create a flat lid while still being able to see what you're doing. If you squint, you risk applying product to wrinkles or folds. For lower eye application, do just the opposite: put your chin down (make a double chin) and look up into the mirror. You'll be amazed how much easier it will be to see your application.

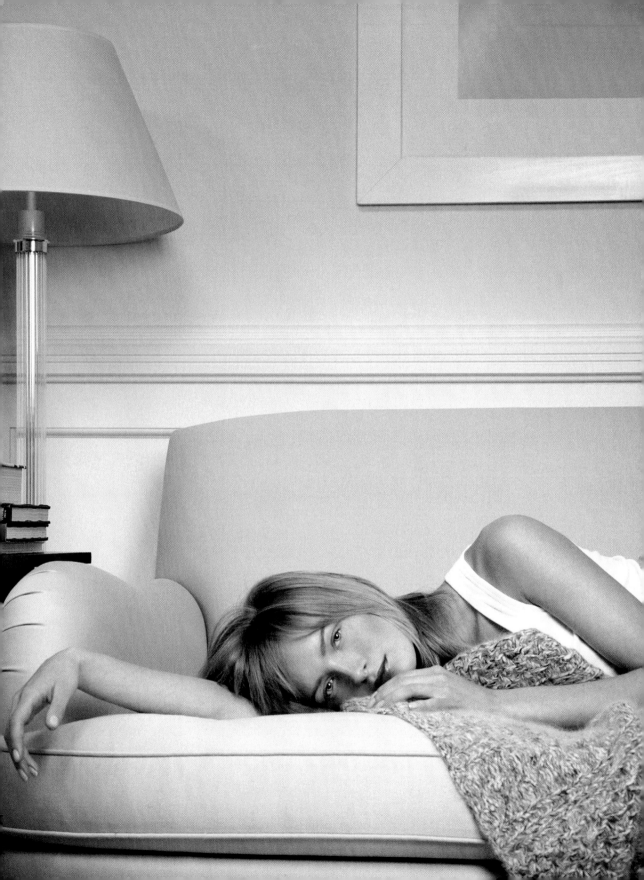

LEVEL ONE

To meet your specific needs, zero in on what concerns you most.

SKIN

REMEMBER THE FOUR STEPS YOU LEARNED IN SKIN CARE—CLEANSE, EXFOLIATE, MOISTURIZE, AND PROTECT. AS A LEVEL ONE, YOU WANT YOUR SKIN TO LOOK ITS BEST.

Options for Coverage

TINTED MOISTURIZER

IF YOUR SKIN IS OTHERWISE IN GREAT CONDITION, A TINTED MOISTURIZER WITH AN SPF OF 15 IS THE CHOICE FOR YOU.

Selection: Pick one as close to your skin tone as possible.

Application: Take an amount that equals about the size of a nickel and apply to the center of the face. Start on your nose and move out across the cheekbones. Blend out with fingers or sponge.

FOUNDATION

IGNORE ANY MISCONCEPTIONS YOU MAY HAVE. IT DOESN'T TAKE A LOT OF TIME TO ACHIEVE GREAT RESULTS WITH FOUNDATION, AND IT DOESN'T HAVE TO LOOK CAKEY OR THICK.

Selection: Choose your color by applying a sample near the jawline. The color should disappear. If you can, try it on in natural light, the best test of all.

Application: Once you have the right shade, assess your skin and apply only where needed—not all over the face. Apply with fingers, brush, or sponge. For best results, start at the center of your face and blend outward. I find it always good to finish blending with a damp sponge or puff to avoid lines of demarcation.

POWDER

FOR ME, IT'S A MAKEUP ESSENTIAL. QUICK AND EASY TO APPLY.

Selection: Pick a powder that matches your skin tone either in place of foundation or to complement it.

Application: Your choice is loose or pressed. Each can be applied with a puff or a full-headed fluffy powder brush. Remember, a brush gives the least coverage. If you use a puff, wrap it around your forefinger like a hot dog in a bun. Press and roll onto skin. Whichever your tool choice, start in the center of your face and blend outward.

CONCEALER

Selection: To hide undereye darkness, pick a shade slightly lighter than your skin tone. Consistency matters: the creamier the texture, the less coverage you'll get. The drier it is, the more coverage you'll receive and the longer it will last.

Application: Use your ring finger to apply concealer, then pat and press.

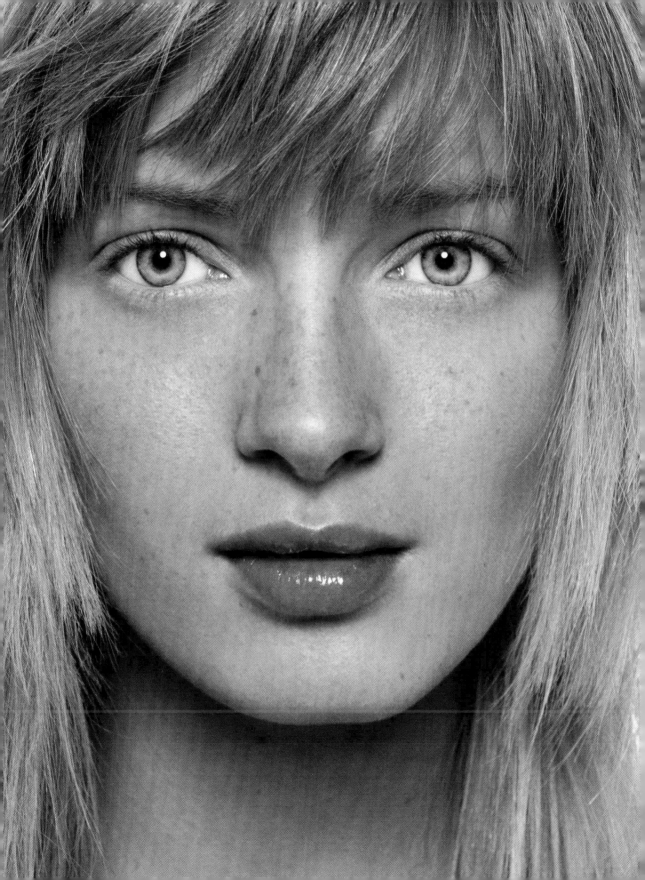

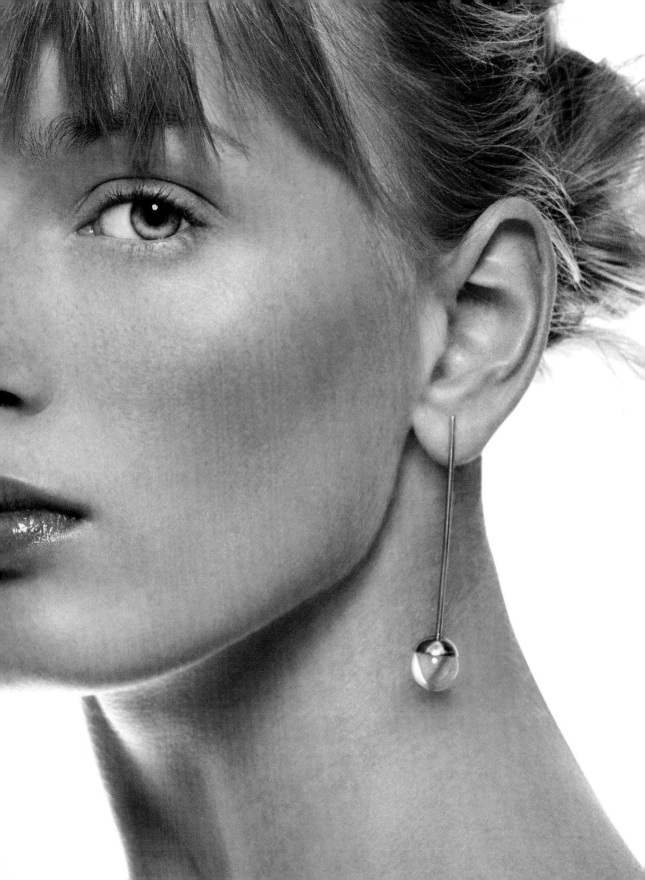

COLOR

If, as a Level One, you want to bring color back to your complexion, you have two choices: blush, which will brighten you up, or bronzer, which will warm you up.

BLUSH

YOU WANT TO LOOK AS IF YOU JUST CAME IN FROM THE COLD (FLUSHED OR SLIGHTLY ROSY) OR AS IF YOU JUST GOT BACK FROM THE BEACH (SOFTLY GLOWING). IN EITHER CASE, MIMIC NATURE IN BOTH COLOR AND APPLICATION.

Selection: Pinch your cheek and the right color will reveal itself. Need more of a color guideline? The darker your skin, the more pigment you may have in the product. I love fair skin in sheer pinks. Medium, olive, and darker complexions are suited to rose tones, apricots, and reds.

Application: It depends on the texture you choose. For all the options, smile and observe the apples of your cheeks. That is where you want to apply the blush. Don't go too close to the eyes or nose (keep at least two fingers away!) nor should you go too low, which can look unnatural and make a thin or small face look gaunt. For balance, add a touch (truly just a touch) of blush to your temple. Always take your puff and blend.

GEL AND CREAM BLUSHES. I like to use fingers. Start at the apple and make a few dots. Blend in a circular motion.

LIQUID BLUSH, STAINS, AND TINTS. Here again, use fingers. Apply product directly to prepped skin. Because it's a stain, you need to work quickly. The good news is that it lasts all day. Remember to wash your hands after application to prevent the tint from staining your fingers.

POWDER BLUSH. Depending on the amount of color you prefer, the brush of choice will make a difference. Remember: the longer the brush hair, the sheerer the application. Also, the first place a brush touches is where you will get the most color. Tap off excess product before it touches your face. Apply blush directly to the apple of the cheek.

BRONZER

WITH BRONZER, YOU WANT MORE OF AN ALL-OVER EFFECT, AS IF THE SUN HAS KISSED YOUR FACE.

Selection: The goal is to look sunny and natural. Pick a color that simply warms up your skin. The fairer your skin, the lighter your bronzer should be.

Application: Feel your cheekbones. Make a C from your cheeks to your temples. When using a powder, use a long-haired bronzing brush. Remember to apply a touch of bronzer under the neck area to make the application look more natural.

OPTIONS FOR LIPS

MOST LEVEL ONES WEAR SOMETHING ON THEIR LIPS, EVEN IF IT'S JUST CLEAR BALM. ON THE OTHER HAND, THERE'S THE LEVEL ONE WHO USES LIP COLOR TO DRESS HER FACE. THAT'S WHY, TO ME, LIPSTICKS ARE LIKE SHOES: THEY CAN EITHER DRESS YOU UP OR DOWN.

Selection: Lip color is personal; pick a shade you love and feel comfortable wearing. For a casual look, go sheer or glossy. If you want a dressier look with a bit more pigment, consider the options of a sheer cream, cream, glaze, or lip/cheek tint. And for even more dramatic lips, go for a semi-matte opaque.

Application: The sheerer the color, the more mistake-proof it will be. If you like more definition and pop, use a pencil to enhance and shape. A quick way to dress up a sheer lip? Fill in lips with the lip pencil.

OPTIONS FOR EYEBROWS

BROWS FRAME THE EYES AND THEREFORE ARE EXTREMELY IMPORTANT TO YOUR OVERALL LOOK. THERE ARE MANY REASONS WHY YOU MAY WANT TO WORK ON YOUR BROWS: PERHAPS YOUR HAIR IS LIGHT OR GRAY, YOU OVERTWEEZED YOUR BROWS IN YOUR YOUTH, THEY HAVE NO DISCERNIBLE SHAPE, OR THEY ARE UNEVEN. FORTUNATELY, IT DOESN'T TAKE MUCH TO BEAUTIFY THEM. YOU CAN IMMEDIATELY SEE THE DIFFERENCE TO YOUR FACE WHEN BROWS ARE CLEARLY DEFINED BY BEING EITHER LIGHTLY FILLED IN OR PROPERLY SHAPED.

Shape: First, make sure your brows are properly groomed. The basic guideline for determining the proper shape is this: hold a pencil against the side of your nose. Where the pencil hits your brow is where the brow should begin. Still pressed against the corner of your nose, swing the pencil to the outer corner of your eye. Where the pencil meets the brow is where the brow should end. Look straight ahead, and the spot above the pupil should be the brow's high point. I like slanted-tip tweezers because they give you the best grip and make it easier to pull in the direction the brows grow. Tweeze from underneath the brow, but whatever you do, don't go overboard. Undertweezed is always better than overtweezed!

Define: If you're happy with their shape after tweezing but still wish your brows looked stronger, maybe all you need is a colored brow gel. Pick a color that closely matches your natural hair color and apply to brows. The gel will groom and color your brows to perfection. If your brows are sparse and you want to fill them in and enhance their shape, you need either a pencil or powder, depending on your preference. If you choose a pencil, use quick, feathery strokes and be sure to follow up by blending with a brush. (I make my eyebrow pencils out of hard lead because I find it creates a more natural-looking brow. I also attach a brush for blending.) If you use powder, apply with a stiff, angled eyebrow brush. Analyze your brows. Where you are most sparse is where you should first place the color.

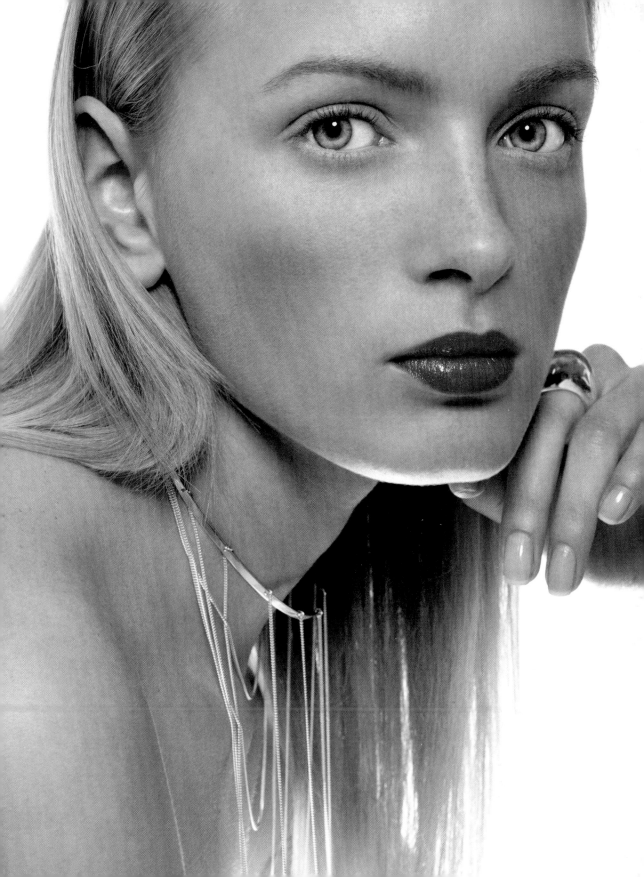

OPTIONS FOR LASHES

CURL TALK

IF YOU DO NOTHING ELSE TO DRESS YOUR EYES, CURL THE LASHES. IT'S THE QUICKEST, MOST NATURAL WAY TO OPEN EYES. ONCE YOU SEE THE DIFFERENCE IT MAKES, YOU'LL BE A CONVERT. (USE THE CURLER FIRST, AND THEN APPLY MASCARA.) I'M AN EVERYDAY CURLING GIRL MYSELF.

Selection: I designed my curler so that the cushion is rounded, not square-edged; it fits right in the curve of your eye socket. Also, the grip is tight and gives you great tension—essential if you want the curl to last.

Application: Tilt your chin up, position the curler's open mouth as close as you can to the base of your lashes, making sure you get the very end ones in. Squeeze. Count to ten and let go.

MASCARA

MASCARA IS THE SUREFIRE WAY TO MAKE LASHES LOOK LUSH AND EYES MORE CAPTIVATING.

Selection: Look for formulas that give quick results without a lot of layers. I designed my mascaras according to clients' needs: Lengthening formulas are for women who want longer lashes. Volumizing mascaras or lash builders are for those whose lashes are sparse. Curling mascaras take up where the curler left off. And waterproof speaks for itself. You can also layer mascara types to get multiple benefits.

Color: Black is the most dramatic, whereas brown gives a softer lash. Or you could opt to have some fun by trying a colored mascara.

Application: First wipe the wand tip with a tissue. Sweep top lashes on the underside from the base to the tips. If you're blond or gray, make sure mascara reaches the base of lashes to hide the color contrast. Wiggle the wand from side to side a bit to ensure more coverage. Make sure you separate and coat outer lashes, too. I'm often asked about applying mascara to bottom lashes. My answer is always the same: it's a matter of personal preference.

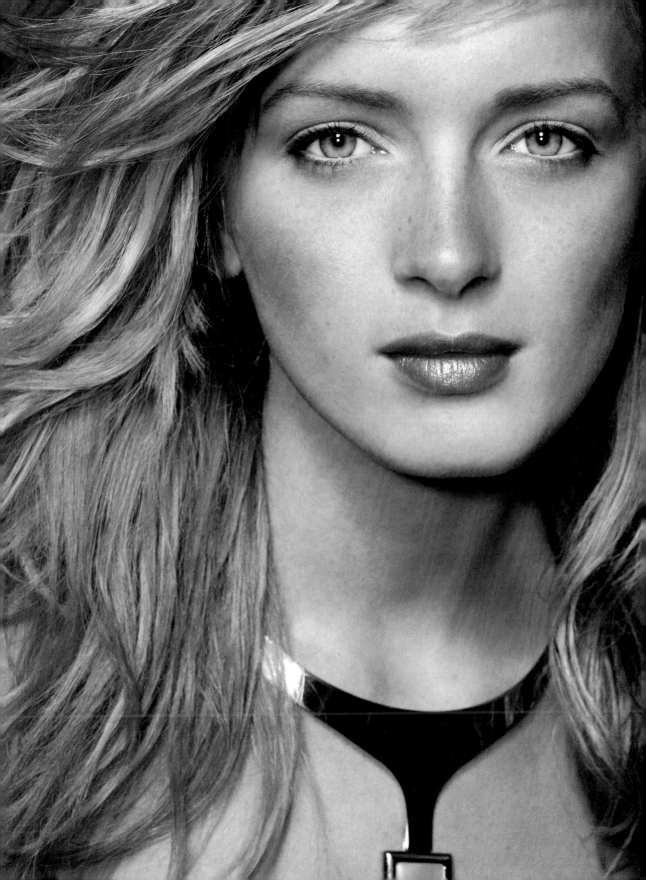

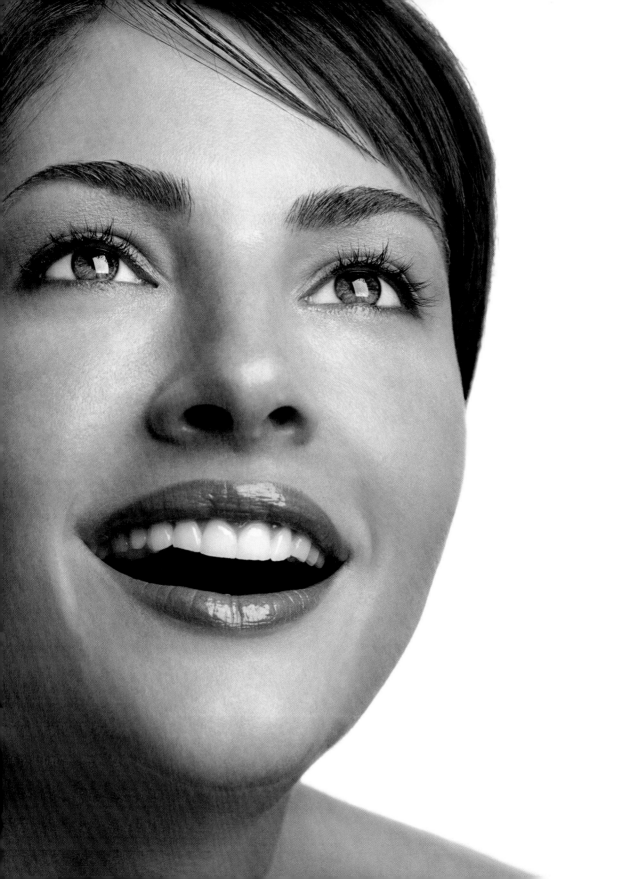

LEVEL TWO

If anything separates you from a Level One, it's your approach to eye makeup.

EYES

IF ANYTHING SEPARATES YOU FROM A LEVEL ONE, IT'S YOUR APPROACH TO EYE
MAKEUP. LEVEL TWOS RARELY FIND EYE MAKEUP OPTIONAL. WE LOVE THE
ENHANCEMENT THAT EVEN THE SIMPLEST EYE APPLICATION CAN GIVE.

Preparation
Apply your eye cream under your eyes and let it be absorbed by your skin.

Shadow Base: This is a product that gives longevity to your base eye color. Holding
your chin up, looking down with your eyes open, you will be able to see the entire
eyelid. Using a laydown brush apply a small amount of shadow base to the entire
eyelid. (I specifically designed my brushes to pick up just the right amount of
product and to fit different eye shapes.) In a pressing motion, apply to the lid,
then use a gentle sweeping motion to blend. Blend up from lashes to brow.

Eye Brush Basics: There are many kinds of eye shadow brushes to choose from, all of
which perform different functions and give different effects and depths of color.
In general, longer bristles will give a wash of color. The shorter the bristles, the
more concentrated the application. Simply put: longer equals less definition;
shorter equals more.

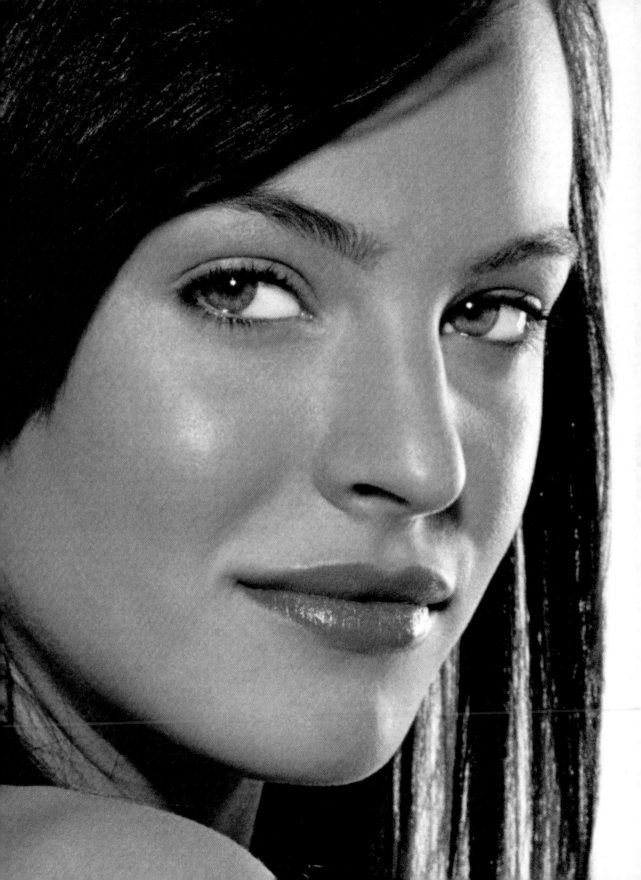

SHADOW: THE CLASSIC EYE

THE KEY TO SUCCESSFULLY APPLYING EYE SHADOW IS TO REMEMBER THE BASIC
PRINCIPLE OF LIGHT AND DARK; LIGHT BRIGHTENS AND BRINGS FORWARD; DARK
RECEDES AND ADDS INTENSITY AND DEFINITION. THERE ARE ENDLESS WAYS TO
MAKE UP YOUR EYES, BUT I'M GOING TO FOCUS ON WHAT WE CALL "THE CLASSIC
EYE," WHICH IS A COMBINATION OF THREE SHADOWS: A BASE COLOR (LIGHT),
A CREASE SHADOW (MEDIUM), AND AN EYELINER (DARK).

BASE EYELID SHADOW

Selection: The color should be a light neutral tone. The color you choose should offer
some coverage.

Application: Remember that your chin should be up, eyes down, lid flat but slightly open.
Dipping your laydown brush into the shadow, apply the light tone to your entire eyelid
from lash line to brow bone. For extra coverage and longer wear, be sure to press and
pat powder into the lid. For lighter coverage, sweep across the lid.

CREASE EYE SHADOW

Selection: This should be a medium tone to enhance the crease area of the eye.

Application: You have two options.
A. *For a soft wash of color,* take a tapered blending brush, dip into shadow, tap off excess
onto a tissue, and place brush on the outer corner of the brow bone. Work inward.
Then blend back and forth in a windshield wiper motion.

B. *For a more defined crease,* take a brush with shorter, tighter hairs, such as my precision
contour brush, dip into shadow, tap off the excess onto a tissue, and press color on the
outer corner of the brow bone. Work inward. Blend back and forth in a windshield
wiper motion.

UPPER EYELINER

Selection: Liner can either be a shadow or an eye pencil.

Application:
A. *Shadow liner:* Take a stiff, thin brush such as my precision eyelining brush and dip it
up and down into your eyeliner shadow. Remove the excess with a tissue. With your
chin up, looking down, start at the outer corner of the eye, placing your brush on top
of your lashes, keeping the brush handle parallel to your cheek. Press and wiggle along
the lash line.

B. *Eye pencil:* Take your eye pencil, hold it as you would any other writing utensil.
With your chin up, looking down into the mirror, draw a line as close to the base of
the lashes as you can, working from inner to outer lashes.
TRISH TIP: *Few women have a perfect, steady hand when it comes to eyeliner application.
Placing your elbow on the dresser table will help a lot.*

AS WITH MASCARA, LINING YOUR LOWER LID IS A MATTER OF PERSONAL PREFERENCE. I DO IT BECAUSE IT GIVES MY EYES MORE DEFINITION, AND I THINK I NEED ALL THE DEFINITION I CAN GET.

Selection: In general, you want to go softer under the eyes. Either use what's left on the brush from applying your upper lid eye shadow or choose a slightly softer tone. For example, if you use black on the upper lid, use a more charcoal tone underneath. Eyeliner shades that have a touch of sheen look especially great under the eyes.

Application:
A. *Shadow liner:* To line the bottom, hold your chin *down* (I mean down; make a double chin), and look up into the mirror. Apply your eyeliner color with your brush, starting at the outer corner of the eye, placing the tip of your brush under your lower lashes. Gently press and wiggle along the lash line. You can make the lower lid clean and crisp, or you can add a little intensity by giving it a subtle smudge. For a smokier application use the same brush as above to apply the line and follow up with a small detail brush such as my precision or soft smudge brushes to subtly smudge it out.

B. *Eye pencil:* Hold your eye pencil as you would any other writing utensil and, beginning at the outer corner of the eye, draw a fine line under the bottom lashes.

LASHES
SO MANY CHOICES HERE—VOLUMIZING FORMULAS, CURLING FORMULAS, WATER-PROOF FORMULAS. THINK OF WHAT YOU WANT TO ACCOMPLISH AND THEN CHOOSE. CURL AND APPLY MASCARA AS I EXPLAINED FOR LEVEL ONE. AS A LEVEL TWO, YOU MAY WANT TO ADD MORE MASCARA TO GET AS FULL A LASH AS POSSIBLE.

EYEBROWS
DOCTOR YOUR BROWS BY FOLLOWING THE APPLICATION IN LEVEL ONE.

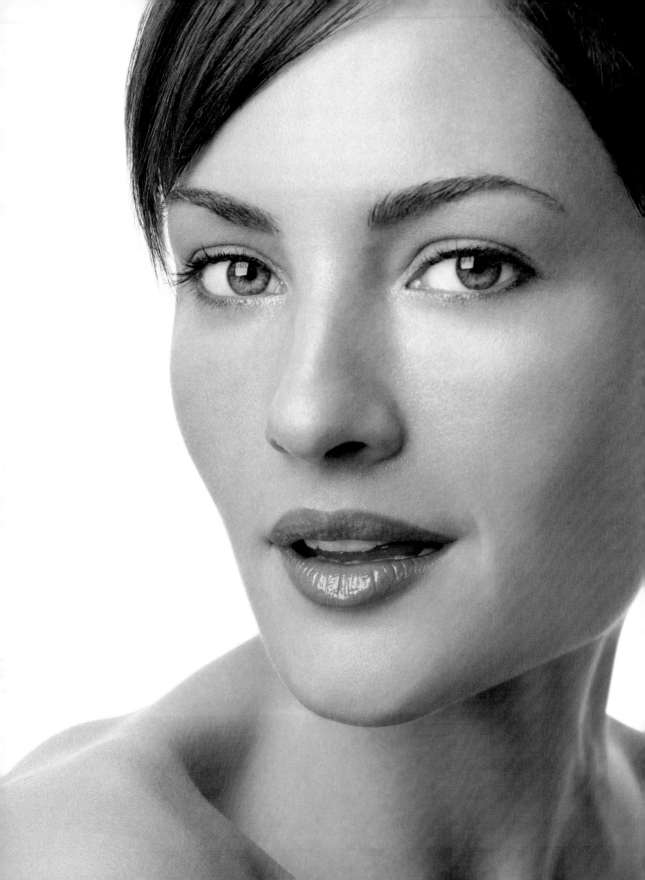

CLASSIC EYE

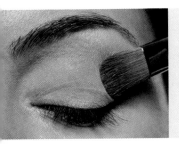

1. Using a large shader brush, apply shadow base, then base eye shadow color in a light tone.

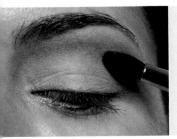

2. Apply crease contour in a medium-toned shadow with a tapered blending brush.

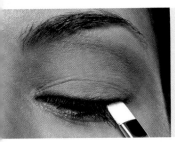

3. Using a flat eyeliner brush or pencil, line the upper lash line with deep-toned shadow.

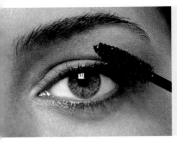

4. Curl upper lashes. Apply mascara.

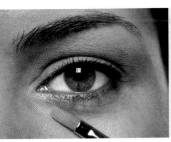

5. Using detailed concealer brush, apply concealer where you are dark. Pat to blend.

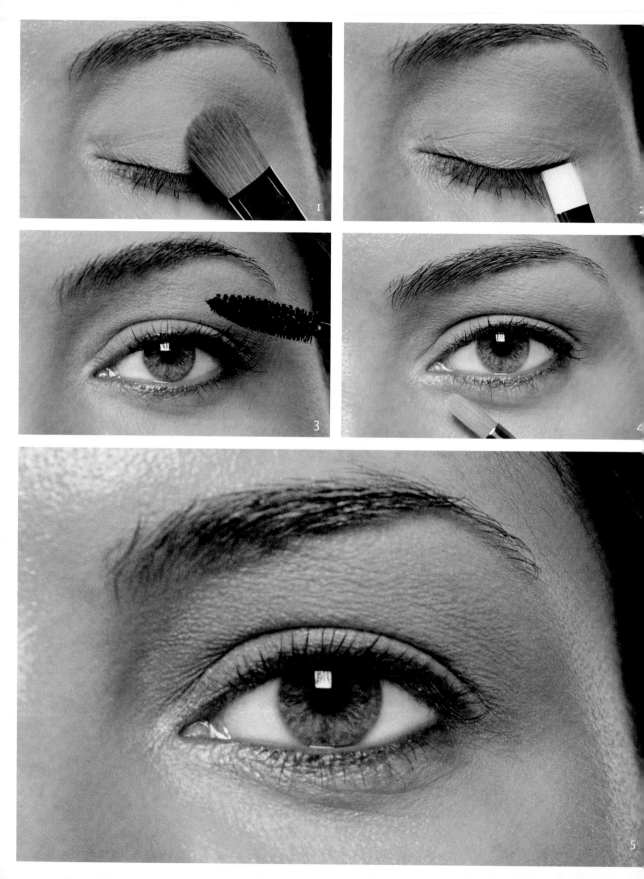

TWO VARIATIONS ON THE CLASSIC
WHILE THE CLASSIC EYE LOOKS GREAT ON EVERYONE,
I HAVE TWO FAVORITE ALTERNATIVES.

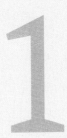

NUDE CLASSIC: *light lid, lined lashes*

Skip the crease color and just wear a light lid and line your eyes as usual.
The look is clean and easy and really opens up your eyes.

1. Using a large laydown brush, apply shadow base to entire eyelid and follow with base eye shadow in a neutral light tone with shimmer over entire lid.

2. Line upper lash line with precision eyeliner brush or pencil using a deep-toned shadow.

3. Curl lashes, then apply mascara.

4. Using a precision concealer brush, apply concealer where you're dark. Pat and press to blend.

5. Finished look.

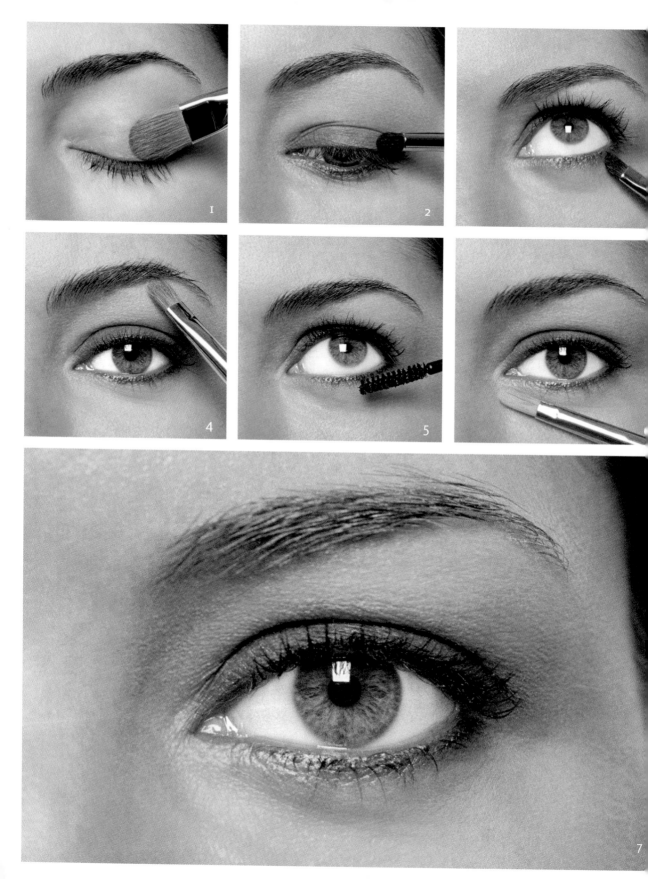

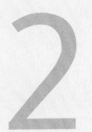

2

SMOKEY CLASSIC: *darker lid, lighter brow bone area*

1. Using a large laydown brush, apply shadow base to entire lid. Follow with light neutral-toned eye shadow over entire lid.

2. Apply medium to dark-toned shadow over ball of the eye using a deep contour brush. Blend over entire eyeball.

3. Use a precision smudge brush with medium to dark-toned shadow. Apply under bottom lashes. Blend back and forth until desired intensity is achieved.

4. Use a small laydown brush. Apply shimmer shadow under brow.

5. Curl lashes. Apply mascara to upper and lower lashes.

6. Using precision concealer brush, apply concealer where you're dark. Pat and press to blend.

7. Finished look.

SKIN: THE PURSUIT OF PERFECTION

BEFORE YOU APPLY ANY FACE MAKEUP, TAKE A SECOND TO LOOK IN THE MIRROR TO MAKE SURE YOUR UNDEREYE AREA IS FREE FROM EXCESS EYE MAKEUP. IF NECESSARY, CLEAN IT WITH A COTTON SWAB AND A TOUCH OF EYE MAKEUP REMOVER AND REAPPLY EYE CREAM.

PRIMER

This is a fairly new innovation that can really affect the look and wear of your foundation. A primer has light-reflecting properties and creates an ideal canvas by sealing in moisturizer and smoothing skin. Apply after moisturizer and before foundation. Start in the center of your face around your nose and work outward. Be sure to let the primer become fully absorbed before you apply foundation.

FOUNDATION

Selection: What does perfect skin look like to you? Does it look moist and glowing? Is it more matte? As discussed in the previous chapter, texture is everything. The perfect finish starts with your prep. If your skin is dry, you should lay the groundwork with an enriched moisturizer, let it be absorbed, and look for a foundation that has some slip to it. If your skin is dry and you want luminosity, take the additional step of mixing your luminizer with your foundation. If you have oily skin and want a matte finish, prep with a mattifying lotion and follow up with an oil-free foundation.

Like most makeup, foundation is highly personal. Some women wear only one particular foundation and consider it a security blanket. Others have a wardrobe of foundations, different finishes for different occasions—perhaps tinted moisturizers for casual days, liquid formulas for everyday, and cream-to-powder for extra-coverage days. All of these approaches are fine. Foundation application is also a matter of preference. Some women swear by fingers, others by brushes, and still others by sponges; many, like myself, may use some combination.

CHOICES

Liquid Foundation. Comes in moisturizing as well as water-based formulas. I like to use the back of my hand as a palette for many things, including foundation. Using a cotton swab, I take just a little, with the idea that I can always add more. Apply foundation with fingers, a sponge (damp or dry), or a foundation brush. For detail work, you can use a large laydown brush.

Cream-to-Powder. Creamy makeup in a compact. Use a sponge, finger, or brush. Dab, press, and blend.

Dual Finish (Wet/Dry). A combination of foundation and powder. Can be applied either dry or with a damp sponge.

Application: Start applying your foundation where you want the most coverage. For most women, that means the center of the face. Start with your nose and work outward. Seldom do you need foundation all over the face. Don't forget to apply foundation around the lips to clean up the area and prep for your lipstick.

LUMINIZERS

Selection: Luminizers are used to brighten your skin. They add radiance or a pretty glow. Luminizers can be used to define your cheeks and can be anything from lighter foundation or powder tones, face shines, or shimmery powders.

Application: Apply directly on the cheekbones. Depending on the texture you choose, blend with either your finger, a sponge, or a luminating buffer brush.

CONCEALER

I LIKE TO APPLY CONCEALER AFTER FOUNDATION.

Selection: When it comes to concealer, it's good to have options, which should include different textures for different areas and purposes. Creamy concealers are great for days when you are not too dark under the eye area; a drier concealer offers more opaque coverage under the eye and is great for uneven pigmentation or blemishes. Having two shades of concealer on hand will save you time in the end, as you can custom match your skin tone and all the variations that can happen day to day with your skin. By mixing two shades, you can expertly create the color you need. For this reason, as well as for convenience, I package my concealers with companion complementary shades.

Application: For strategic placement you want to use a small pointed brush such as my precision concealer brush. This will allow you to get into corners and other hard-to-reach areas and let you place your concealer exactly where you want coverage. For general blending, look to brushes such as medium or large laydown brushes. The best concealer brushes come in nylon or sable. Pay attention when you apply concealer. Really look at your skin and see what kind of concealer the area calls for. Colorwise, you want to match your skin as closely as possible, with the exception of under the eyes, where you want to go one shade lighter.

TRISH TIP: *The key to concealers is to keep building (adding additional layers) until you have the coverage you want.*

POWDER

I CAN'T SAY IT ENOUGH. NEXT TO BLENDING (WHICH POWDER HELPS TO DO), POWDERING YOUR FINISHED FACE IS THE ONE RULE THAT BEARS CONSTANT REPEATING. AFTER ALL THE TIME YOU'VE SPENT ON APPLICATION, YOU WANT YOUR MAKEUP TO STAY EXACTLY HOW AND WHERE YOU PUT IT FOR AS LONG AS POSSIBLE. POWDER MAKES THAT HAPPEN. TO ME, POWDER IS THE CLOSEST THING YOU HAVE TO MAKEUP INSURANCE.

Application: Depending on the coverage you desire, you can use a puff, sponge, or brush. A puff will deliver more powder for more coverage; a damp sponge lets you turn dual powder formulas into foundation. A brush delivers the sheerest application—just the right amount to finish and set the foundation or to even out bare skin tone. Whichever you choose, dip the applicator into the powder and remove the excess. Apply over entire face except for areas where you do not desire a matte finish.

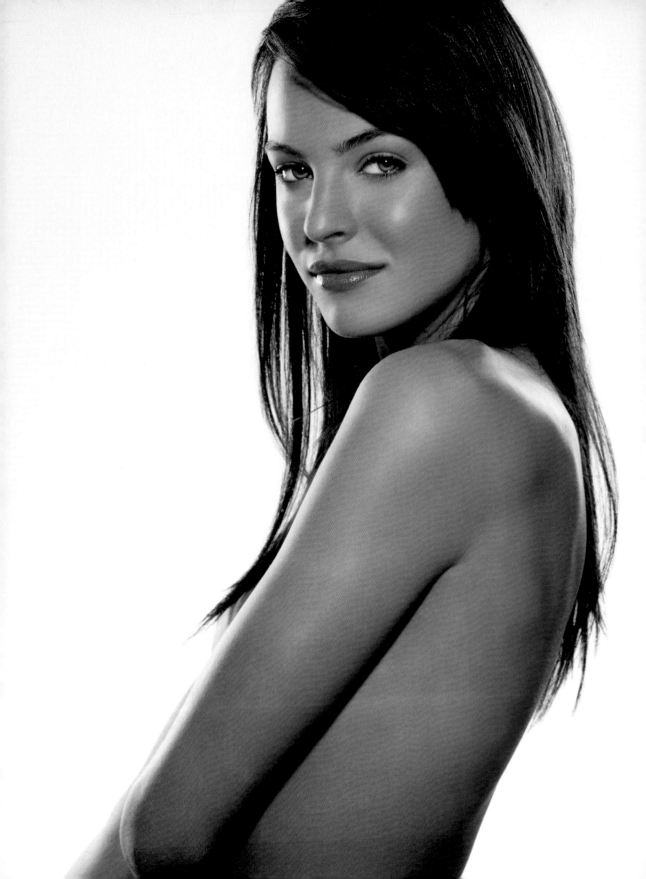

COLOR

ALMOST EVERYONE BENEFITS FROM THE UPLIFT OF COLOR OR BRONZER. COLOR
IMITATES GOOD HEALTH AND YOUTH. CONSIDER HOW CHILDREN ALWAYS HAVE
THAT ROSY FLUSH. THE GOAL WITH COLOR IS TO RECAPTURE THAT GLOW.

Selection: As I described in Level One, you can opt for blush or bronzer. For a more
dimensional look, you can wear the two together or add shimmer.

Application: Make a C shape from the cheeks to the temple with bronzer. Blend.
Sweep a dot of a brighter toned blush onto the apples of the cheeks. Blend together.

LIPS

YOUR LEVEL TWO STATUS PROBABLY MEANS THAT YOU LIKE YOUR LIPS A BIT
MORE DEFINED THAN YOUR LEVEL ONE SISTER. A FEW STEPS CAN HELP YOU
APPLY LIPSTICK LIKE A PRO.

Selection:
1. Lipstick is about choice of color and texture. Remember, a shimmer will make your
lips look fuller (great for thin lips) and a semi-matte is one of the dressiest (perfect
if you choose to make your lips the focal point of your face). You may also experiment
with mixing colors and layering textures—for example by placing a dot of shimmer
in the center of a semi-matte lip.

2. A serious lip gal will always opt to line her lips. I like liner colors that are in the
same family as your natural lip color. A natural color will clearly define your lips,
be versatile, and never overpower the lipstick you're wearing.

TRISH TIP: *Choose a lip pencil that glides easily (not too hard, not too soft) onto the lip.
Keep pencils sharpened.*

Application: To get the best results, prep properly. Lip balm will keep your lips in good
condition. If your lips have fine lines or are thin, use a product that addresses that
concern. In applying foundation around the lips, you help the lip liner or lipstick do
its job by creating a cleaner line. Starting where the pigment of your lip begins, use
the side of your lip pencil to trace your natural lip shape. Fill in with your lipstick.
Don't worry if you make a mistake. Just blot down the color and reline the lips.

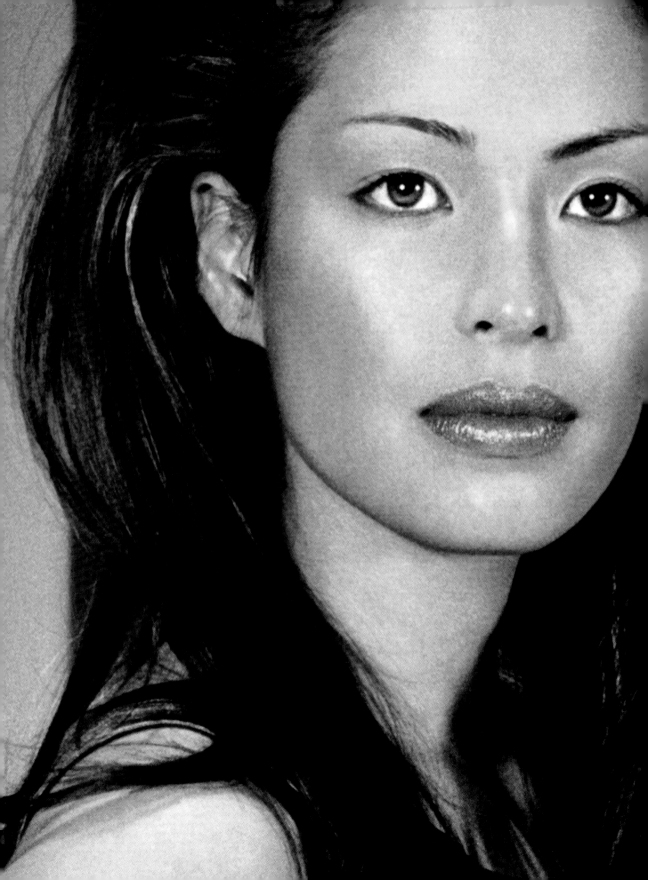

LEVEL THREE

*If eyes separate a Level Two from a Level One, then it's the intensity
with which you apply makeup to whatever feature you want to
emphasize that separates you from a Level Two.*

EYES

IF EYES SEPARATE A LEVEL TWO FROM A LEVEL ONE, THEN IT'S THE INTENSITY WITH WHICH YOU APPLY MAKEUP TO WHATEVER FEATURE YOU WANT TO EMPHASIZE THAT SEPARATES YOU FROM A LEVEL TWO. THE TECHNIQUES ARE THE SAME. BEGIN YOUR APPLICATION THE SAME WAY AS YOUR LEVEL TWO SISTERS. CREASE COLOR MAY BE MORE INTENSIFIED; PERHAPS YOU MAY ADD A TOUCH OF LUMINOSITY TO THE INNER CORNER OF THE EYES. YOUR LINER MAY EXTEND FURTHER IN OR OUT ALONG THE LASH LINE AND MAY ALSO HAVE MORE DEPTH OF COLOR.

TRISH TIPS:

1. *Highlight the inner corner of the eyes by using a glazed eye shadow or shimmery pencil to follow the eyes' natural inner V.*
2. *For the ultimate in definition, consider using a liquid liner or wetting your cake eyeliner.*

FALSE LASHES

I THINK FALSE LASHES CAN BE AN OPTION IF YOU WANT A FULLER LASH LOOK.

Selection: The most natural (and also my preference) are the individual lashes. The strip kind are more dramatic. The individual lashes are like hair extensions, and the strip is like a fall. Colorwise, I find a mixture of brown and black looks best. Whichever you go with, have them professionally trimmed or experiment with trimming them yourself.

Application: First equip yourself with your supplies—cuticle scissors to trim, tweezers to apply, the lashes, and the glue. Squeeze a small dot of glue onto the back of your hand. Using tweezers, pick up a lash (or strip) and dip its end into the glue. Give it a chance to dry a little before you place it. Adhere a false lash to the base of your natural lashes. Continue until you create the fullness you desire. Apply mascara in several light coats to seal in the false lashes with your own.

Removal: Put a dab of eye makeup remover on a cotton swab and dab at the base of lashes. Gently pull them off. Then remove the remaining glue, as well as any mascara buildup, with makeup remover.

TRISH TIP: *False lashes take dexterity, patience, and practice.*

EYEBROWS

DOCTOR YOUR BROWS BY FOLLOWING THE INSTRUCTIONS IN LEVEL ONE.

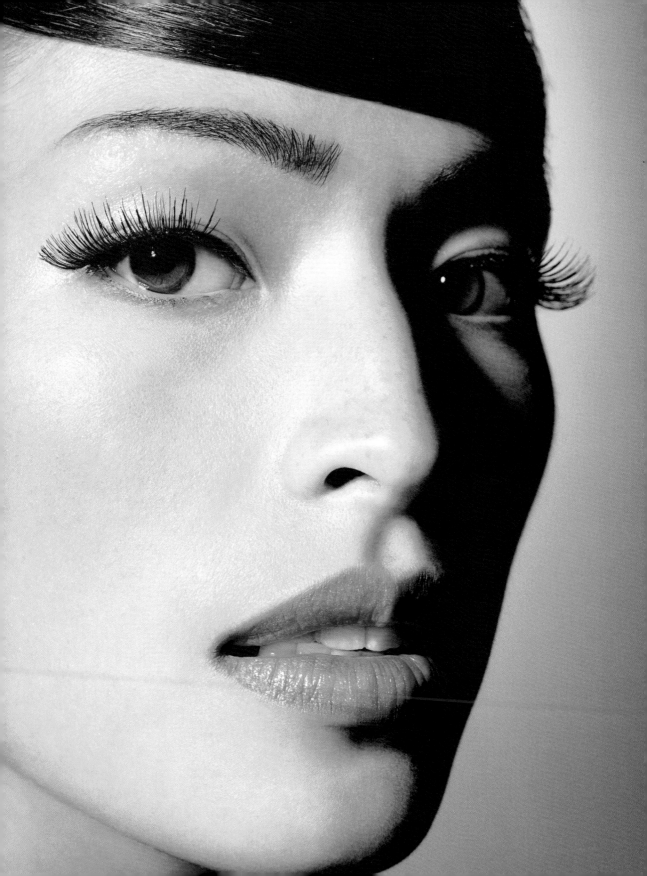

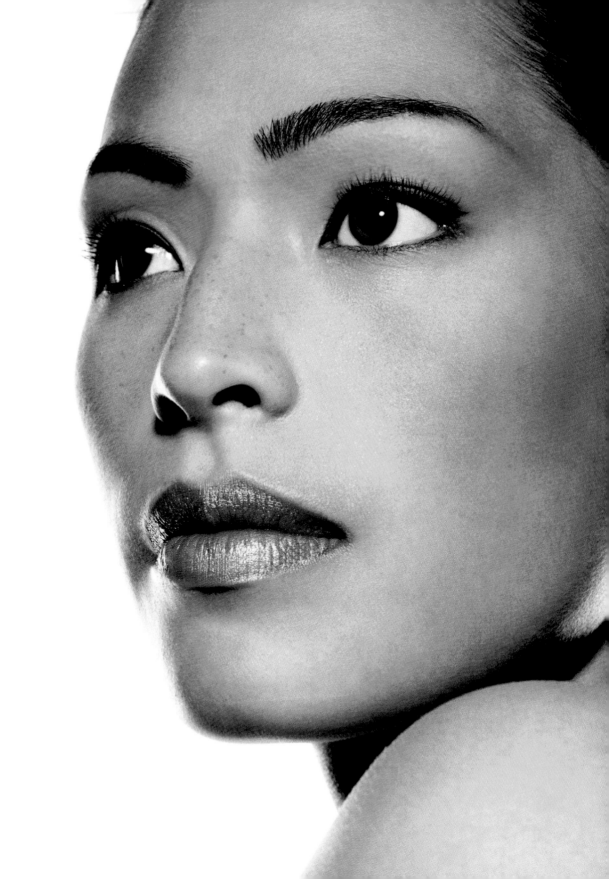

SKIN

EVERY WOMAN I KNOW WOULD LOVE TO HAVE PERFECT SKIN. AS A LEVEL THREE, YOU WILL DO WHATEVER IT TAKES TO ACHIEVE A FLAWLESS LOOK AND FINISH.

FOUNDATION
Pick a texture and color that suits your skin—the better your skin, the sheerer your texture. Apply foundation as discussed in Level Two.

SHADER
Used to bring out the structure of your face. The flip side of a highlighter, it can be a slightly darker foundation or a darker face powder. (The one thing it can't be is a luminizer or any product with a shine, because you want the area to recede, not come forward.) Apply along the lower side of the cheekbone, in a slight curve up to create the most natural illusion. Blend the edges of the shader with a clean brush, puff, or sponge. There should be no lines of demarcation.

CONCEALER
Every face, whether young or old, appears fresher with a strategic application of concealer—and not just under the eyes. Use on areas of your face that require more coverage than foundation alone. With a precision concealer brush, apply a tiny amount of concealer to any small blemishes you want to hide. Press and pat to blend with either your finger or a cream detail brush.

POWDER
As we already have discussed, powder will set your makeup. For more coverage, load up your puff by pressing it into the loose powder. Now press the puff onto the back of your hand to see how much you have. If you like the amount, apply in a rolling motion onto your face. For a sheerer finish, use a sponge or a powder brush, as previously discussed, and sweep across your skin.

COLOR
No matter what your Level, looking healthy is important. Cheek color gives you that glow. To achieve a look that best suits your style, choose your color and texture, and follow the steps outlined in Level Two. This step comes after highlighting and shading.

LIPS

You need to decide if you want your lips to be a focal point in terms of color. Whatever your decision, you will need to spend time to make your mouth look its best on your finished face. A lip brush is a must to help ensure a perfect shape. After applying lipstick, take a cleanup brush, dip it into your powder, and place powder along the outer edges of the lip. Buff excess powder away with a wedge sponge.

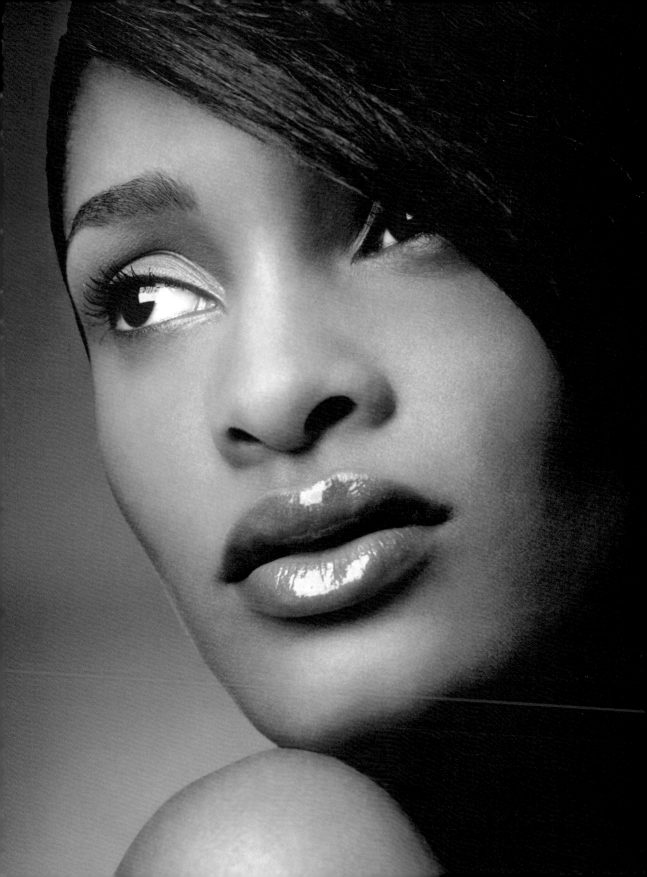

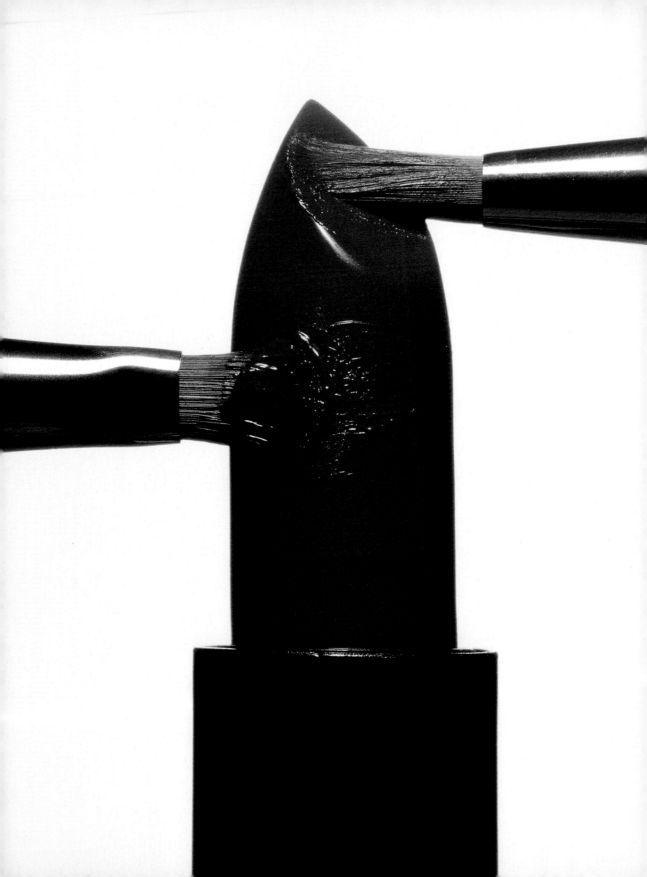

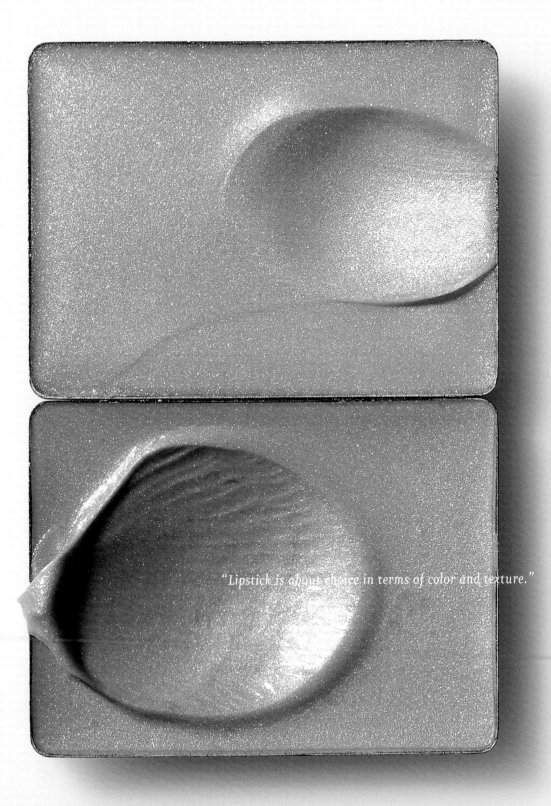

"Lipstick is about choice in terms of color and texture."

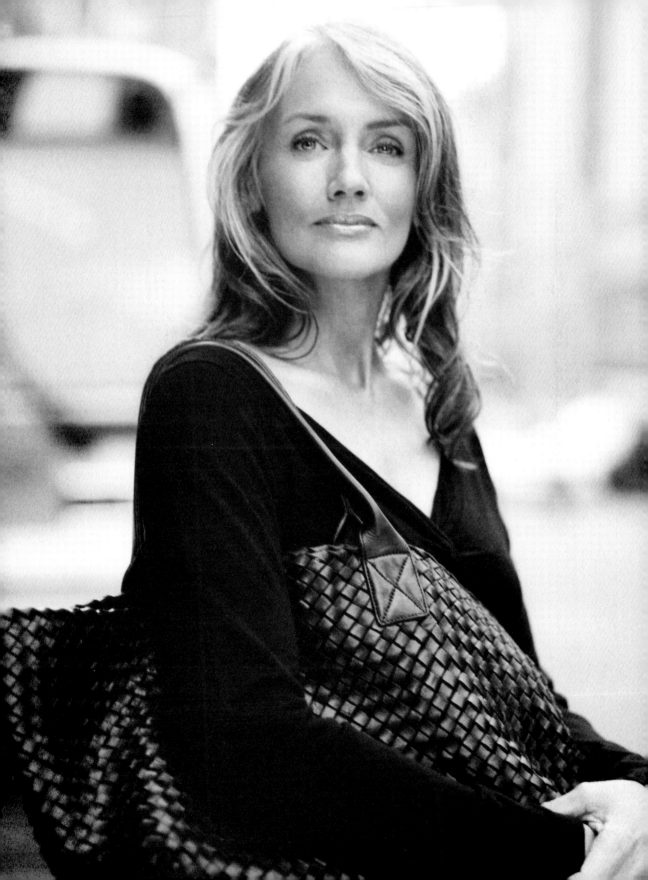

THE AGE FACTOR: *Making the Right Adjustments*

7

I'M GOING TO TALK ABOUT GROWING OLDER WITHOUT USING ANY NUMBERS. HERE'S WHY: WOMEN DON'T AGE ACCORDING TO NUMBERS. MY MOTHER-IN-LAW IS NINETY-FOUR BUT LOOKS A GLAMOROUS SEVENTY-FOUR. I'VE WORKED ON THIRTY-YEAR-OLDS WHO LOOK FORTY AND FORTY-YEAR-OLDS WHO LOOK TWENTY-FIVE. WE EACH HAVE A VISUAL AGE THAT MAY OR MAY NOT CORRESPOND TO OUR CHRONOLOGICAL ONE. WE ALL MAY SHARE COMMON AGING PATTERNS, BUT YOUR PARTICULAR ISSUES MAY SURFACE BEFORE OR LATER THAN THOSE OF A FRIEND WHO HAS THE SAME BIRTHDAY. IT WOULDN'T BE ACCURATE TO GIVE YOU MAKEUP SUGGESTIONS BASED ON A NUMBER.

How young you look is determined by many factors; some are in your control and some are not. The factors you can't control are your genes. The factors you can control include sleep, your current diet, a religious use of sunscreen, and some makeup tricks. Makeup, that trusted pal, can really help you look fresher and younger.

There are benefits to getting older. I had a rounder face when I was young and have been delighted by the angles and cheekbones that have since appeared. One important thing that comes with age is confidence. You've grown into your looks. You've moved on from all the questionable makeup experiments of your youth and know what doesn't work.

Age is as much a state of face as it is a state of mind, and your face is just not as predictable as it was when you were twenty. A twenty-year-old, for example, looks pretty much the same whatever the circumstances. She can have a late night but wake up looking refreshed with no circles under her eyes. She can forget to exfoliate, yet always have a glow. Advancing years, however, change all that. Try going to bed at three in the morning and not seeing it on your face the next morning. It's almost impossible. Conversely, a weekend at the beach will probably make you look rested, and you'll glow with less help from makeup. Remember, if you're good to yourself, you'll look good. It's that simple.

Of course, few of us have stress-free lives in today's world. There are days when you just look older due to circumstances out of your control. I know this myself. I recently went away on a business trip to train my makeup artists. There was so much to fit in and not enough time, and I wanted to do everything. So I did what many women do: I cheated on sleep and kept pushing myself forward. But then came that moment when I looked into the mirror and realized that the week had caught up with me.

Unfortunately, the moment came on a day I'd be spending with clients. I knew I had to make up for those late nights and early mornings. At that point I had to evaluate what needed extra help. I pulled out my Planner and magnifying mirror and got to work.

For many of us, that morning look into the mirror is the critical moment of the day. You look at your reflection and decide if you're happy with what's looking back. If you are, you proceed with your normal routine. If your face needs something, it will communicate that need. If your skin looks dry or dull, it's asking for extra moisture, to be exfoliated, and maybe to be treated to a luminizer. If your skin looks unusually colorless, a blush or a bronzer is in order. If you're looking at darkness around the eyes, you want to reach for an eye cream with light reflecting qualities and expect to spend more time with your concealer. If your foundation isn't going on well, your skin may be requesting exfoliation. Pay attention and respond accordingly.

One of the myths I hear all the time is that an older woman should wear less makeup. What you may really need is more strategically placed makeup. I say "may" because I don't believe there are any absolutes. If you look in the mirror and are happy, then just smile. There's no cosmetic in the world that can compete with bliss. For those off days, however, I have some suggestions. Use as needed.

Today is the youngest you will ever be. Enjoy it!

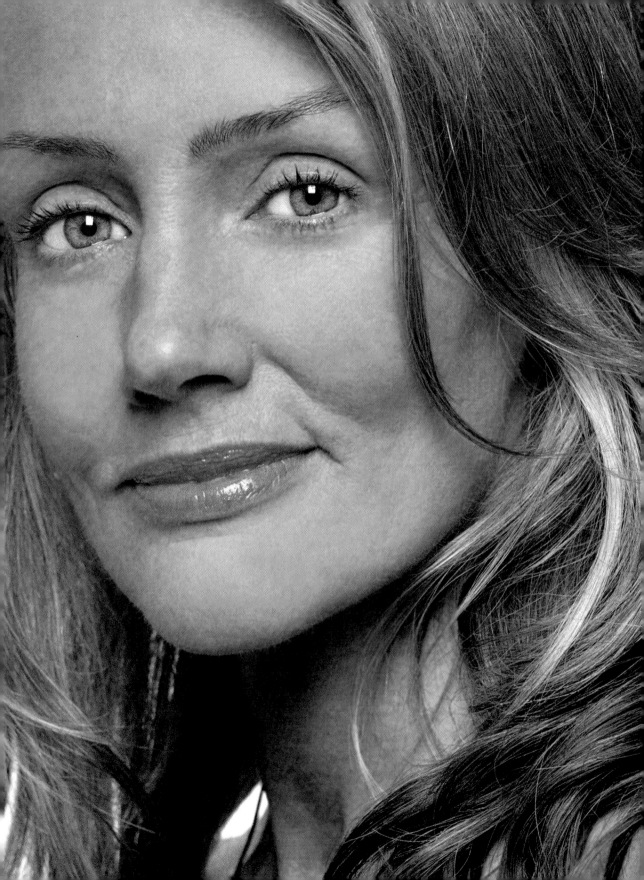

FACING THE FUTURE LEVEL BY LEVEL

Unless your lifestyle or makeup preferences change, there's no reason to leave your Level as you age. Yet, there are basic adjustments that can benefit most women whatever your look and style. For example, adding luminosity brings back the glow that may have faded over time. Defining your eyes and addressing sparser eyebrows can really make a difference to the overall impact. And when it comes to skin, coverage and evening out pigmentation become more important. My suggestion is to work on anything that bothers you, yet consider at least trying the other tips I offer as well. You may be delighted by what just one extra step can do. Your Level will determine how much time and energy you're willing to invest. As these pictures show, there is more than one way to age gracefully.

AGING CLASSIC EYE

1. Apply neutral cream shadow to base of eyelid.

2. Blend with fingertip from base of lid up.

3. Using a precision eyeliner brush, line close to upper lash area.

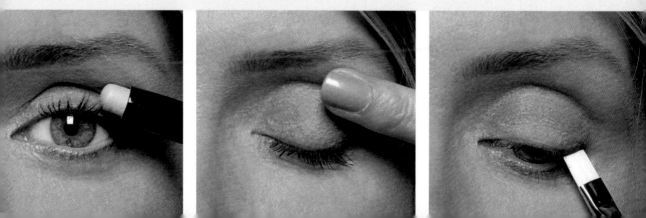

EYE "LIFTS"

Issue: The skin around your eyes looks tired and dry.
Solution: This is a common one. Skin seems thinner, and fine lines are more noticeable on the eyelids, near the corners (crow's-feet), and under the eyes. Arm yourself with an eye cream, preferably one with reflective properties. Prep skin and wait for it to dry. Then apply foundation and concealer.

TRISH TIP: *Heavy eye makeup not well blended can make you appear older.*

Issue: Your eyes look a little droopy.
Solution: Defy gravity! Upswept lines, a slight tilt of the eyeliner at the outside corners, a higher arc of crease color, and a wash of highlighter along the brow bone, just under the brow, can help create the illusion of a new shape.

TRISH TIP: *Skin-tone eye shadow choices can make you appear younger.*

Issue: Your eyelashes and eyebrows seem lighter and sparser.
Solution: As you get older, hair gets grayer (or whiter) and can become thinner, too. (Alas, it also becomes thicker where you don't want it.) Thinning hair can occur anywhere, from the top of your head to your lashes and brows. For lashes, you may want to go to your local salon and have them dyed a darker shade. But that won't make them thicker. To plump up the lashes, you may want to consider a volumizing mascara. For brows, this may be the time for some enhancement by way of powder or pencil. Even if you've never touched your brows before, this is the time to at least think about it, especially if you've started coloring your hair. (See page 128 for defining eyebrows.)

SKIN ENHANCERS

Issue: Your complexion is uneven.
Solution: As you get older, you may find that you have uneven pigmentation (including a shadowy nasolabial fold) from all those years of being in the sun. Creating the look of younger skin is less a matter of hiding wrinkles than of relying on a little extra coverage to even out your skin tone. Foundation and concealer help lighten the dark areas and make your shadows less noticeable. You may also want to apply concealer on your eyelids to reduce darkness as well as the appearance of veins.

Issue: Skin has lost its glow.
Solution: It may be just temporary or a continuing trend that I call "fading." In any event, you want to put back your old glow. You need to exfoliate, use a moisturizer enriched with light reflective qualities, and add a luminizer. This is a case in which a little more is better than a little less.

TRISH TIP: *When applying foundation, mix in a little luminizer for an added boost.*

Issue: My blush just doesn't look right.
Solution: Colors that mimic nature will make you look more rested. Placement is key. Keep the blush on the apple of the cheek, not too low, and use a brush that will allow a gentle sweep of color.

TRISH TIP: *Natural-toned blushes will make you appear younger and more rested. Darker tones can add years.*

Issue: You've gone gray, and your usual makeup seems too harsh.
Solution: Whenever you change your hair color, gradually or otherwise, you need to adapt your makeup colors. If you've gone grayer or whiter, you'll want to do two things with your makeup: go softer and make it more defined. The two are not contradictory. Your colors should soften up to complement your lighter appearance; instead of a black liner, you may want to opt for charcoal. You'll want to brighten your cheek and lip color. You'll still want to define your features as much as you can, only use a softer, more gray-friendly palette.

TRISH TIP: *Softer and brighter don't mean lighter.*

LIP SERVICE

Issue: Your lips seem thinner.
Solution: It's one of those simple and aggravating facts: lips thin as we get older. Even Mick Jagger's are thinner now! You may need to define your lips more. For a natural but strong lip, start by prepping your lips with lip balm. Then, using a lip pencil in the same color as your lips, line your lips and then fill them in with the lip pencil. As you apply, really work it in. The lip pencil and the balm will work together to make your lips seem fuller. I also like to apply face powder around the lips both to lighten the surrounding skin and to make sure the balm doesn't move outside the lips.

TRISH TIP: *Try some of the new lip products that have extra moisturizers to plump up lips.*

Issue: Flaking, dry lips get in the way of applying lipstick.
Solution: Take out your toothbrush and gently give your lips a good once-over. Afterward, rub in a balm and apply lipstick as usual. On those days when your lips are drier, pick a sheerer, more moist lip color formula.

TRISH TIP: *Apply lip balm before doing your makeup to allow it time to settle in.*

Issue: Lipstick always seems to travel outside your lip line.
Solution: Line lips with a pencil that closely matches your natural lip color and fill in the lips.

TRISH TIP: *Apply a touch of an antifeathering lipstick base around the outline of the lips to keep lipstick in its place.*

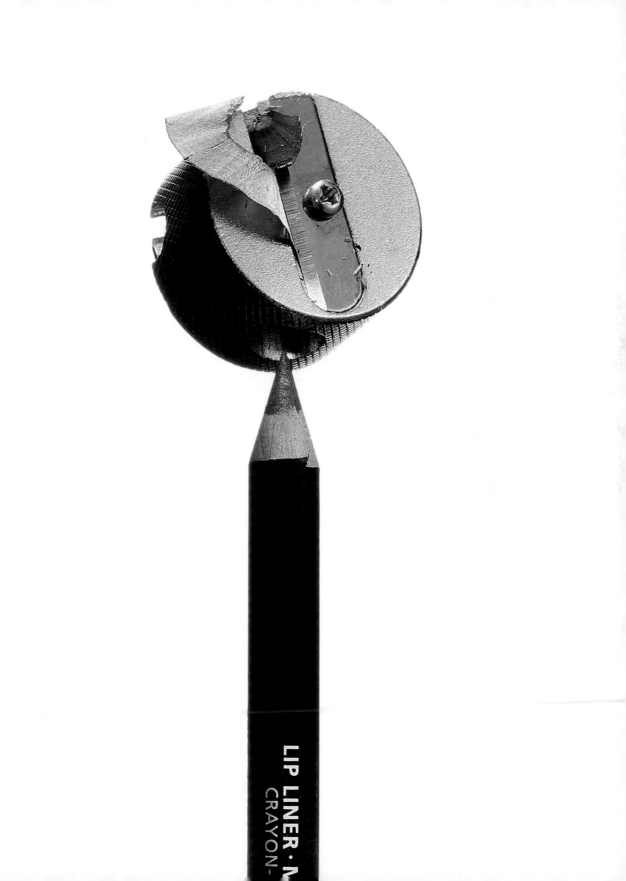

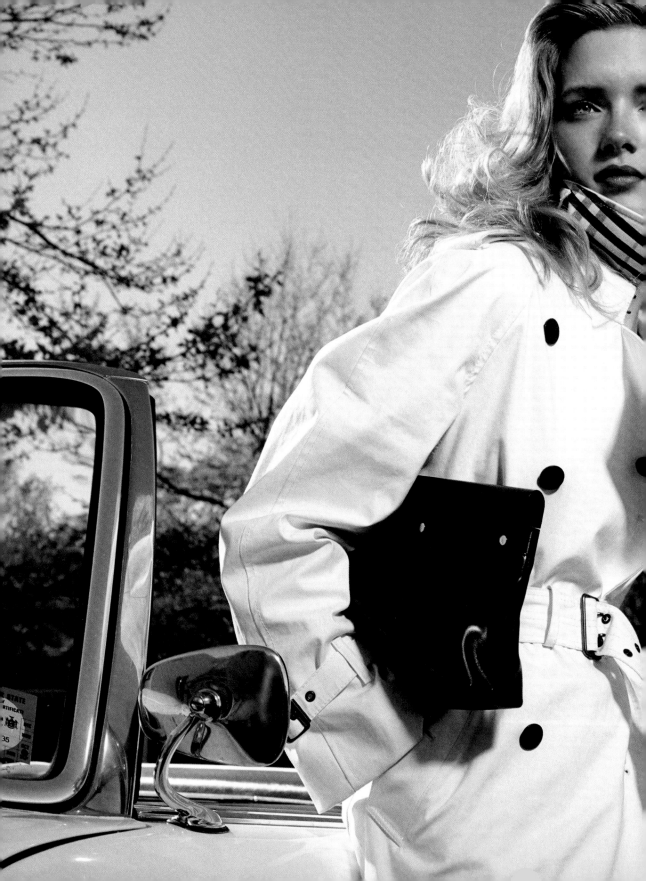

BEAUTY IN MOTION: *Taking Your Makeup on the Road*

IN AN IDEAL WORLD YOU'D WAKE UP IN YOUR OWN HOME EVERY DAY WITH ALL THE TIME IN THE WORLD TO MAKE UP YOUR FACE. YOU'D HAVE THE LUXURY OF THE BEST LIGHTING, YOUR MAKEUP WOULD BE IN FRONT OF YOU, AND YOU'D KNOW EXACTLY WHAT TO DO AND WHAT THE RESULTS WOULD BE. BUT IF YOU'RE ANYTHING LIKE ME, YOU'RE NOT LIVING IN THAT WORLD. TIME IS ALWAYS AN ISSUE, AND REAL-LIFE RESPONSIBILITIES AND SCHEDULE SWITCHES CAN GET IN THE WAY OF THE BEST-LAID PLANS. YOU'RE ON THE MOVE, FROM THE MINUTE YOU WAKE UP TO THE SECOND YOU LIE DOWN AT NIGHT. MY BET IS THAT YOU WOULDN'T HAVE IT ANY OTHER WAY.

I know I wouldn't. I love being busy, and that includes traveling for work and pleasure. Moving around, however, changes anyone's makeup regimen. Climate fluctuations change your texture needs. Then you have to think about the activity at hand, your choice of clothes, and makeup appropriateness. You wouldn't wear stilettos on the tennis court not only because it would look bizarre (to put it mildly), but because the shoes wouldn't function.

There are always beauty constants—the essentials that you need and wear no matter what else is going on. For example, whatever else is going on in my life, I have on an SPF 15 moisturizer, concealer, blush, powder, lip color, and probably mascara, too. For me, that's bare bones. (I told you I wasn't a Level One.)

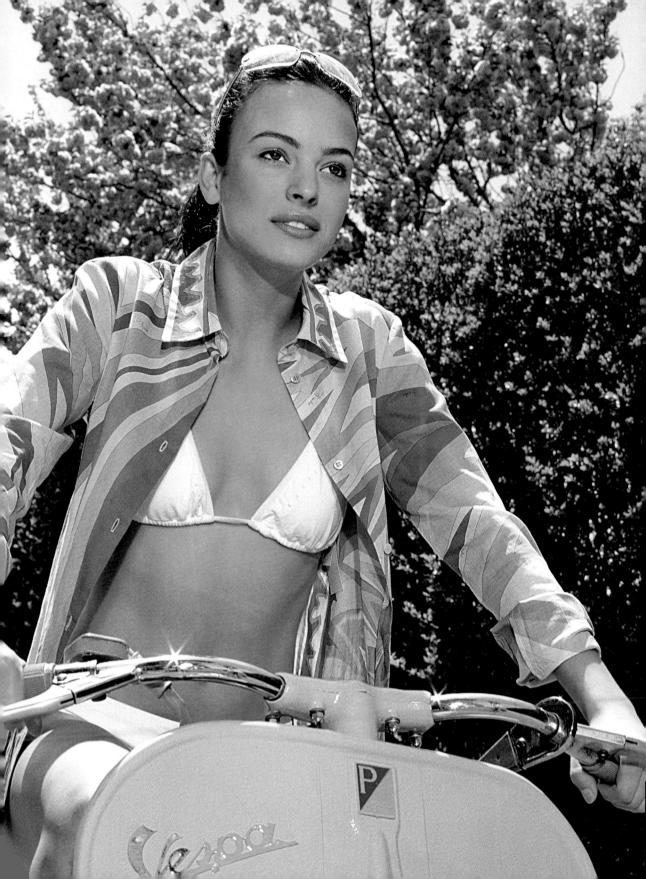

BEAUTY EMERGENCY KIT

EVERYBODY NEEDS A BEAUTY EMERGENCY KIT, WHETHER YOU KEEP IT
IN YOUR OFFICE OR YOUR GLOVE COMPARTMENT. TO ME, IT'S A SECURITY
BLANKET, FULL OF THINGS THAT IN A PINCH CAN BE BEAUTY SAVERS.
HERE IS MY SUGGESTED LIST. NATURALLY YOU MAY WANT TO ADD OR
SUBTRACT, DEPENDING ON YOUR NEEDS.

1. CONCEALER, for days when your undereyes need that extra coverage.

2. BLUSH, for when you need that quick, extra pick-me-up.

3. POWDER, so that they'll never see you sweat.

4. BLUSH/POWDER BRUSH, to give you perfect application every time.

5. PUFF, the great corrector of all makeup mistakes.

6. LIP BALM, perfect for dry-lip days and for applying under lipstick.

7. HAND CREAM, for those days when your hands cry out for it.

8. LIPSTICK/GLOSS, because you never know when you'll need a touch more color.

9. SMALL TUBE OF CORTISONE, for skin emergencies.

10. TISSUES, for the runny days.

11. BAND-AIDS, for new-shoe days.

12. SMALL MIRROR, for the details, darling.

13. FRAGRANCE SAMPLE, if you wear it. I wouldn't go anywhere without it.

14. BREATH MINTS, the quickest way to freshen up.

15. ASPIRIN, because you never know who's going to give you a headache.

16. BOTTLE OF WATER, if you have the space. I like
the convenience of having it with me.

17. EYE DROPS, because you don't want to be caught red-eyed.

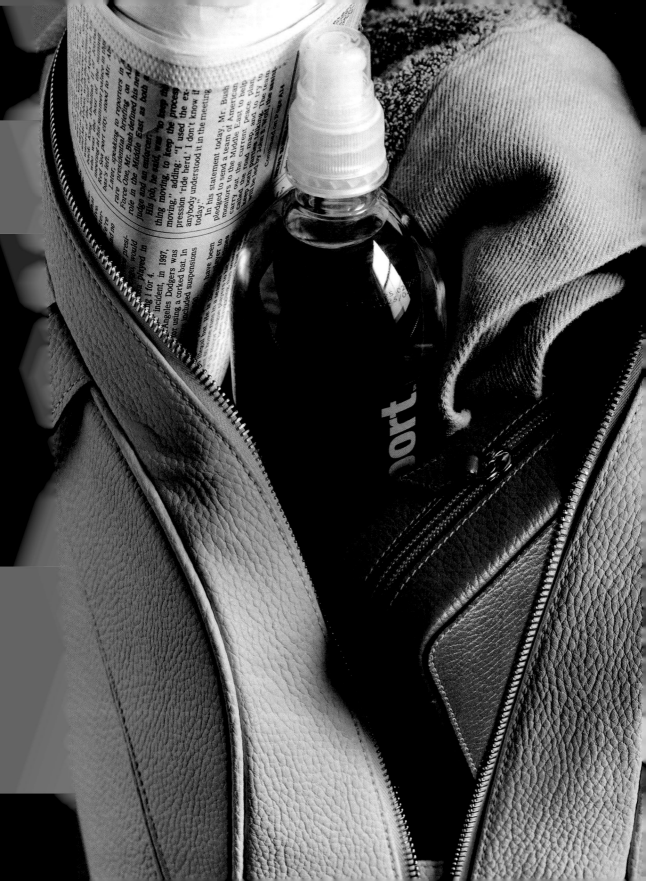

SITUATIONAL STRATEGIES

FOR MANY OF US, LIFE IS LIVED ON THE GO. HOW YOU APPROACH A GIVEN MAKEUP SCENARIO DEPENDS ON MANY THINGS, STARTING WITH YOUR LEVEL. VISUALIZE WHAT YOUR DAY MAY LOOK LIKE AND WHAT YOUR NEEDS WILL BE. PREPARE ACCORDINGLY.

SHORT ON TIME. Women often tell me that if there's one luxury they have had to give up in life's shuffle, it's time to themselves. That means they need to put on their makeup quickly but without sacrificing the results. My biggest suggestion: if you don't already, use brushes to apply makeup—and don't forget the puff. They will cut the time it takes to apply your makeup in half. Also look into using multifunctional products: lip crayons that double as blush, a curling mascara so that you can forget the lash curler, maybe a tinted moisturizer or cream-to-powder foundation. Skip the lip liner (which requires precision) and wear a more forgiving sheer lip color or gloss. You'll be surprised at how much you can accomplish in a few minutes if you have the right tools and products all organized in one place at your fingertips.

THE GYM. Don't wear makeup when you work out. It won't stay on anyway. The time to put your makeup on is after your workout. If you're using the gym's showers, don't take chances on its skin supplies, such as the cleanser and moisturizer. Use only what you know. Bring your usual skin cleansers and shampoos with you, in miniature sizes. If they don't come in small sizes, then purchase the handy plastic dispensers available in most drugstores and create your own miniatures. If I'm heading directly to work after my workout, I'll also bring along my makeup Planner.

A BIG EVENT. This is when you want to look your most special. By all means pull out all the stops. Be sure to schedule ahead for your hair, nails, and facial. When it comes to your makeup, block out a leisurely chunk of time, put on your favorite music, and expect to indulge in all the details. Perfect your skin with the works: foundation, concealer, blush, luminizer, and powder. Also spend the time to put on layers and layers of mascara. But especially, to up the beauty ante, think tactical: maybe you'll want to intensify your eyes with a smudgier effect or choose a more dramatic, dressier lip color.

AT THE OFFICE. In addition to your own beauty emergency kit, it's a great idea to have a duplicate makeup kit in a desk drawer with all your absolutely, can't-live-without makeup. In addition, you should have your favorite skin-care products in miniatures for those times when you need to start from scratch. Also invest in a leave-at-work, good-quality mirror—a big one—for touch-ups. You want to be able to close your door (if you have one) and comfortably apply your makeup much the way you do at home.

OFFICE TO CASUAL. If you're heading to a baseball game after work, you'd probably no sooner keep the same makeup on than you would wear your work clothes. The objective here is to tone it down. If your daytime look includes lined eyes, you may want to smudge and lift some of it off with a cotton swab. (Don't worry, you won't remove all of it.) Take out your puff and blend down your foundation and blush to their barest. And, lastly, take a tissue and keep blotting away at your lipstick until it's just a stain, then add gloss.

OFFICE INTO EVENING. When it comes to evening plans, your preference would be to go home, soak in a tub, and then begin to get ready. Instead most of us find ourselves getting ready in the office bathroom, at a desk, or in a car. No matter, you can do a fine job with just a change of makeup. If you can, wash your face and start from scratch. At any Level, the most important thing when spinning day into night is to add more definition. Ask yourself, where do I want the focus? Lips, eyes, or both? Then apply your makeup to address those areas. Lastly, spritz on some fragrance. For me, scent is the ultimate way to shift moods.

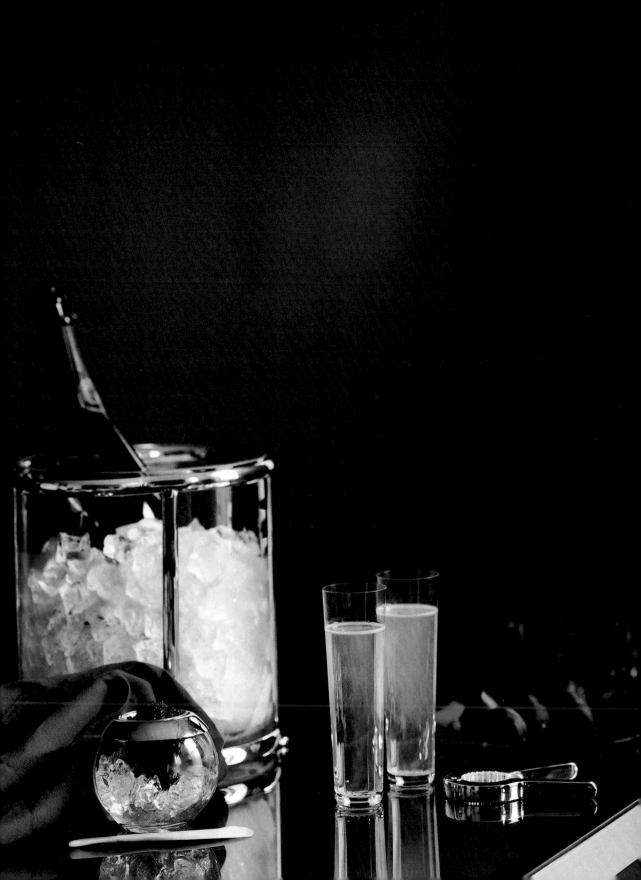

AIRPLANE BEAUTY

UNLESS IT'S A SHORT TRIP (UNDER TWO HOURS), LESS IS MORE FOR AN
AIRPLANE REGIMEN. YOU WANT TO WEAR YOUR BAREST ESSENTIALS: CONCEALER
AND MAYBE A BIT OF LIP COLOR. YOU WANT TO HYDRATE YOUR SKIN AS MUCH
AS POSSIBLE WITH EYE CREAM, MOISTURIZER, LIP BALM, AND HAND CREAM. I'M
ALSO A BIG BELIEVER OF SPRITZING THE FACE. BEFORE THE FLIGHT ENDS, I TAKE
OUT MY PLANNER, APPLY MY MAKEUP, AND I'M READY TO LAND.

ZIP UP AND AWAY

Some pump containers can leak due to pressure changes at
high altitudes. To be on the safe side, store them in Ziploc bags
separate from your other makeup items. Also, be careful with
products in tubes. Pressure changes can make them spurt out
quickly and unexpectedly when you first open them.

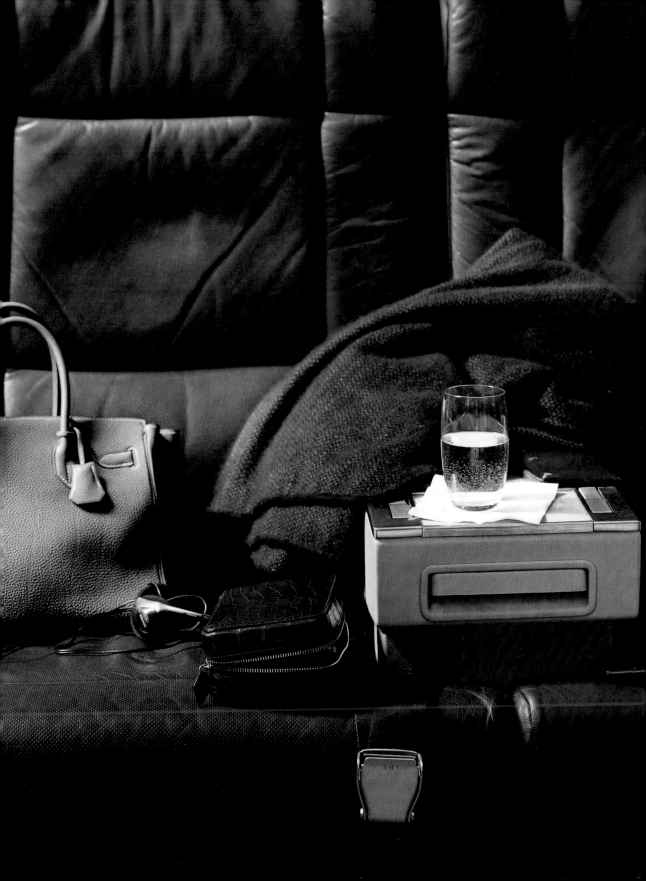

CLIMATE CONTROL

WHETHER YOU'RE TRAVELING TO THE ENDS OF THE EARTH
OR ENDURING DRASTIC TEMPERATURES AT HOME, YOU'LL WANT TO ADAPT
YOUR MAKEUP ACCORDINGLY.

Tropical heat and cold weather enhance your coloring by giving you a natural flush. The first thing you need is an SPF 15 moisturizer. Be generous with the application, and make sure you let it bond to the skin before putting anything on top of it. Remember, if you're in a sunny climate, you are probably exposing more skin, so be extra diligent.

Now that your skin's protected, think of how it will look in glaring sunlight. Even if you're going for a no-makeup look, you may want to even out your skin tone, especially dark undereye circles or any redness around the base of the nose. You'll want to curl and coat your eyelashes with water-resistant or waterproof mascara. And you may want to wear a nude lip pencil with clear balm. Even in the harshest light, you'll look like you're barely wearing any makeup.

Of course, you're not always skiing or swimming when you're in such weather. Sometimes you're in a professional or social situation and you simply want to preserve your usual look. Here are some tips to keep in mind:

EXTREME HEAT

Your goal is not to wilt. To give your look longevity in the face of humidity and triple-digit temperatures, switch to lighter textures and snap up a few products that fend off unwanted sheen. If you're very oily, start with an oil-free, SPF moisturizer that has a mattifier. Or apply an oil-control product to the T-zone of your face. Use a sheer, water-based foundation and/or powder.

EXTREME COLD

Snow and chilly air can give you the beauty boost of a rosy glow. But it can also make your skin and lips drier if you don't adequately prepare. You want to increase your moisture straight across the board. Wear a moisturizer that's at least one degree richer than your usual formula. If you normally wear a lotion, consider a cream formula. Don't skip undereye cream and lip balm. To add a dewy glow to your skin, consider a switch to cream-based eye, cheek, and lip colors. Now's not the time for anything powdery.

"A makeup lesson can be a really good
time if you approach it with a sense of
fantasy and adventure."

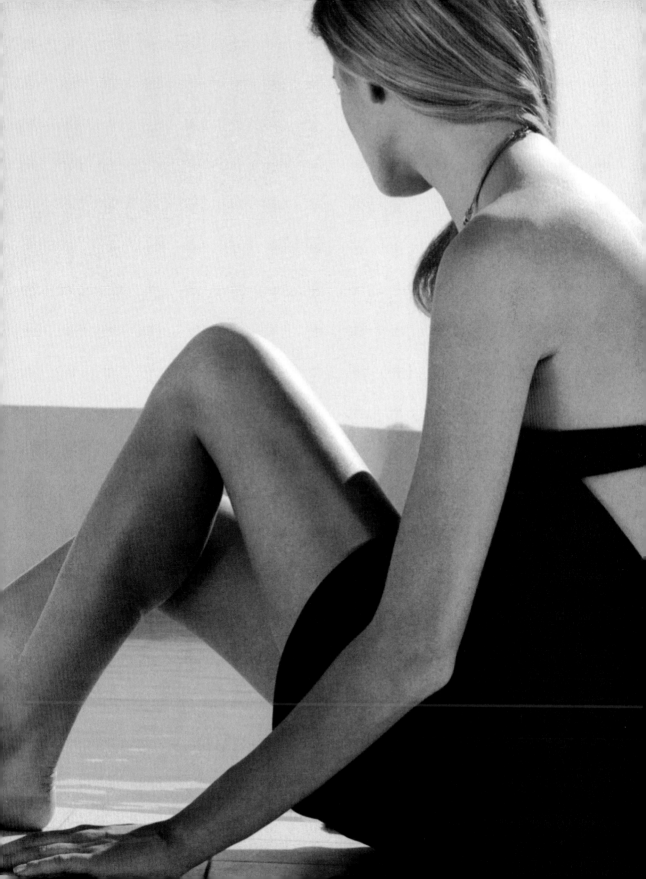

HOW TO SHOP BEAUTY

HERE ARE SOME GUIDELINES TO KEEP IN MIND AS YOU APPROACH A COSMETIC COUNTER. THE MORE PROACTIVE YOU ARE, THE MORE YOU WILL GET OUT OF THE EXPERIENCE.

1. SEEK A MAKEUP ARTIST YOU'LL FEEL COMFORTABLE WITH.

If you love how someone looks, she'll probably have a lot to teach you. But even if she's not quite your style, it doesn't mean that she isn't able to give you what you need. Ask her to describe her own makeup. If she's heavily made up and says it's a "natural" look, that may well be her idea of natural, and you'd be right to question if she's the one to help you (assuming you're after a natural look). Just don't be quick to judge by appearance alone. I have Level Three makeup artists who can do absolute wonders with minimal products for their Level One clients.

2. COMMUNICATE YOUR LEVEL.

Tell the makeup artist the role makeup plays in your life, both in terms of time and style. A Level Two doesn't want a Level Three demonstration.

3. BE OPEN-MINDED.

Experiment. Otherwise you'll never learn anything new. Don't get stuck in a makeup rut. Try new techniques, textures, and color; you never know what will click.

4. STATE YOUR PREFERENCES.

Describe how you like to look. Better yet, bring your favorite picture of yourself. Communicate whether you like matte or shiny, bronze or pale, if you like sheer or strong lips, neutrals or color. Show her the colors you're currently wearing or have in your makeup case. Anything that helps steer the makeup artist to your comfort zone saves you both time and energy.

5. BRING IN PICTURES OF MAKEUP LOOKS YOU LOVE.

This is where magazine tear sheets come in handy. I don't have to tell you how many words a picture can save.

6. SPEAK UP THROUGHOUT THE CONSULTATION.
As you're shown things, express your opinion. If you like something, say so. If it's not for you, a simple "That's not my thing" is fine. Each comment helps the beauty expert to help you better.

7. LOOK AT YOUR MAKEUP IN DAYLIGHT.
This is key! Take a second to walk outside with a mirror. Daylight is the ultimate test, because if it looks great in daylight, it looks great in any light.

8. IF POSSIBLE, TRY ANY NEW APPLICATION TECHNIQUE YOURSELF WHILE STILL IN THE STORE.
I firmly believe that you only learn by doing. My makeup artists are taught to teach you. It's like step dancing; you need to follow along until you can pick it up for yourself. Keep working with the makeup artist until you feel confident you have the technique down. Try to leave the store with written directions so that you don't have to rely on your memory the next day.

9. IF YOU LIKED THE CONSULTANT WHO HELPED YOU, GET HER NAME AND STAY IN TOUCH.
There's a lot to be gained from holding on to a makeup artist you connected with. She'll keep you on file and be familiar with what you like and own. Tell her if you'd like to be called or e-mailed when it's time to replenish something (she can always mail it) or when new products come in. She can also put you on her invitation list to call for upcoming specials and beauty events.

10. GO FOR YOUR PERSONAL BEST AND HAVE SOME FUN.
A makeup lesson can be a really good time if you approach it with a sense of fantasy and adventure. While a makeup artist cannot turn back the clock or turn you into a supermodel, she is trained to help you look your personal best. Whether you want a pull-out-all-the-stops red carpet look or a dewy, natural look, this is the place to experiment and have fun. Don't forget, you can always wash it off!

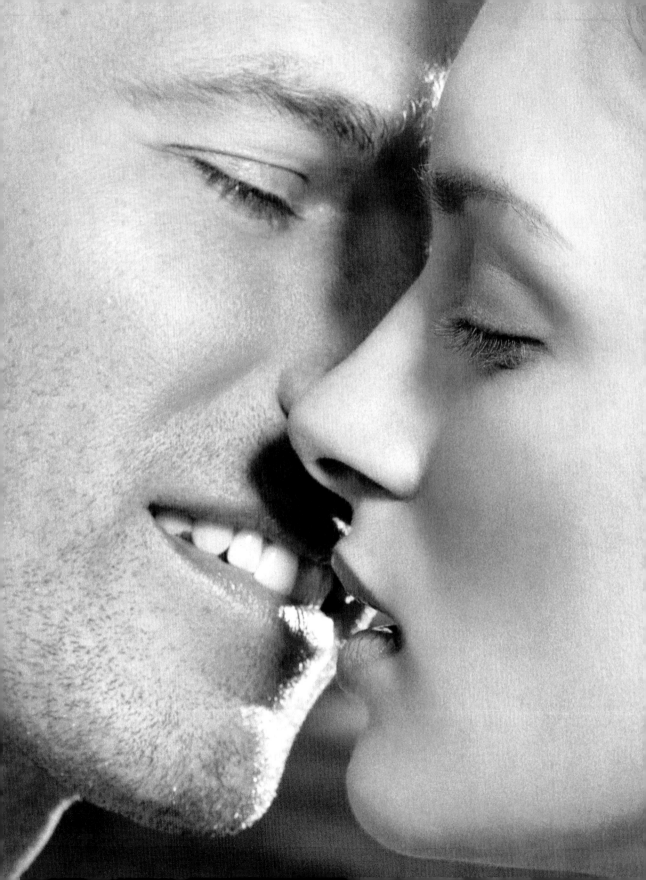

DETAILS, DETAILS, DETAILS: *The Things That Really Matter*

BEAUTY IS IN THE DETAILS. PIECE BY PIECE, IT'S THE DETAILS THAT FILL OUT THE PICTURE AND CREATE THE OVERALL IMPRESSION. ALL THE ELEMENTS HAVE TO WORK TOGETHER TO EXPRESS THE WHOLE. THE RIGHT HAIRSTYLE, AN EVEN COMPLEXION, A HEALTHY GLOW, SEDUCTIVE LIPS, WELL-GROOMED HANDS: THE SUM OF THE PARTS IS A UNIQUE PORTRAIT OF A PERSONALITY—YOURS.

I believe that joy is also in the details. It's the little things you do for yourself that put a smile on your face. With the right detail, you can turn a mundane chore into a pleasure. For example, if you wash your hands with a favorite scented soap, you come away smelling good, and the experience is richer for it. If you use a special pen to jot down notes, writing is more enjoyable. If your handbag has pretty colored accessories, it is a delight to look inside. Use a good or fun-colored umbrella and rain doesn't seem so bad. Wear beautiful lace underwear and you feel beautiful underneath it all. Getting the details right adds ease and happiness to your life. Most of the time it doesn't even take a lot of money, just a little extra planning and attention.

If you don't pay attention to the details, you risk undermining your whole look. As a woman passionate about organization, I believe that you can minimize the time you spend on beauty details, whether you're talking about manicures, dyeing and cutting your hair, exfoliating your body, having facials, picking up flowers or living with fragrance. As much as we love the world of beauty, most of us can't devote our day to it. Life is not a spa, but if you plan it right, it can feel like one.

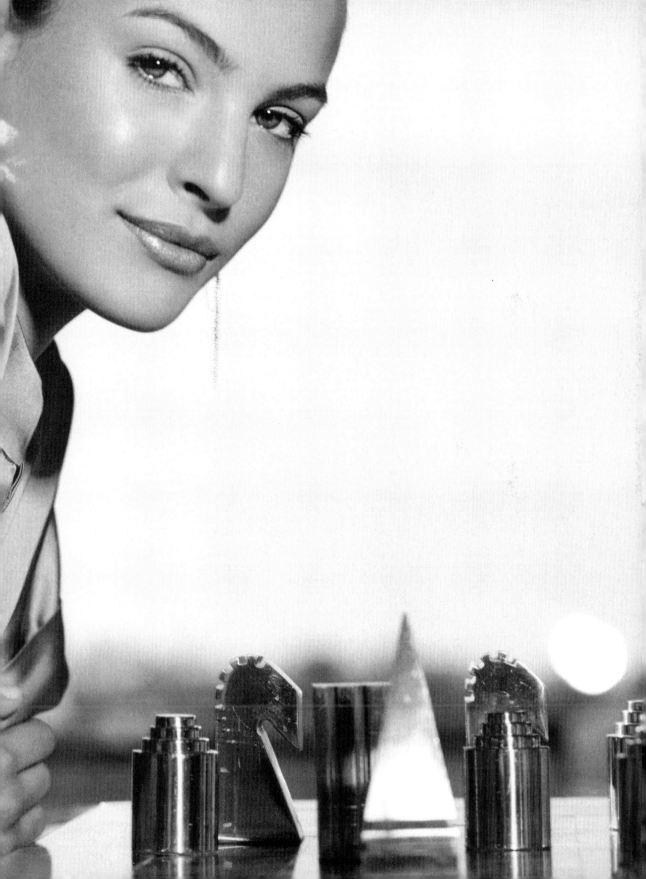

THE FINISH LINE:
HOW TO ORGANIZE THE DETAILS

1. PRIORITIZE.
First things first. Even if you wanted to dot every I and cross every T, you couldn't.
Life's too short. Decide what matters—the nonnegotiables—and commit.

2. PLAN IN ADVANCE.
If you have a big night, book the hair stylist as early as possible and have a facial
a week in advance. If your nails matter to you, have a standing appointment.
Don't wait for cosmetics to run out before replenishing them.
Anticipate what you'll need and when you'll need it.

3. IMPOSE ORDER.
Declutter. Edit your medicine cabinet. Rid your handbag of anything
you don't need. Edit your makeup bag; remove duplicates or items you don't use
and replenish what you need. Have only the things you use in front of you.

4. WHERE POSSIBLE, TAKE SHORTCUTS.

Since time is limited, always ask yourself if there is a faster, more efficient way to do something. This is where dual-purpose products make a difference, such as an SPF moisturizer or a hand and body lotion. One of my favorites is our lip and cheek tint.

5. SIMPLIFY, SIMPLIFY, SIMPLIFY.

The simpler a task is, the more you are apt to do it. Pare down your routine to the fewest steps you can get away with. Do you really need to shampoo twice? How many coats of nail polish are truly necessary? Don't skip what matters, just the superfluous extras.

6. BE CONSISTENT.

The most important advice of all. You know how helpful it is to put your keys in the same spot every day. Whatever the detail is, roll it into your routine so that you won't forget it. You shouldn't have to scramble to remember something important.

FOUR
QUICK FIXES

DESPITE THE BEST-LAID PLANS, YOU'RE BOUND
TO RUN INTO AN OCCASIONAL BEAUTY CRISIS. HERE ARE
SOME IMMEDIATE BEAUTY PRESCRIPTIONS TO GET
YOU THROUGH THOSE TOUGH MOMENTS.

Dilemma: You had a bad night's sleep.

Beauty RX: Focus on lightening any shadowy areas and add subtle touches of brightness to your complexion and lips. Start by blending concealer over dark areas, especially under the eyes and in the nasolabial folds around your mouth. Don't make an arc under your eyes; dab it only and exactly where needed. Add a pop of rosy blush to your cheeks and slip on a slightly brighter, translucent lip color. (Avoid opaques on tired skin.) I also like a light dusting of bronzing powder. Mascara does wonders for opening the eyes, creating the illusion of a wide-awake face.

Dilemma: It's the morning after a late-night dinner or party.

Beauty RX: First, moisturize your skin because you're probably a bit dehydrated. You probably look tired, too. Tempting as it is, don't overcompensate with makeup, because it will only point up what you're trying to hide. If you have dark circles, reach for the concealer and apply directly on the shadows. Add some bronzer or blush to perk up your sallow complexion and consider some sheer lip color.

Dilemma: You woke up to a big, fat, pink blemish.

Beauty RX: If you can get to a dermatologist for a shot of cortisone, it will reduce the inflammation. If you can't get to a dermatologist, whatever you do, don't pick at it. Just forget that idea. Instead put on a drying lotion or medication and be sure to use a cotton swab, and apply the treatment only on the pimple itself. Let the treatment dry. Then take your concealer and apply it with a tiny brush, right on the top of the spot. Work it around in a one-centimeter-wide radius, then take a cotton swab and buff away the edges. Set with a touch of powder. Now comes the hardest part: just forget about it. Really, a pimple is just not worth ruining your day.

Dilemma: It's been a long, tough day, yet you still have two meetings ahead of you.

Beauty RX: Take five minutes and refresh yourself. Step into the washroom and blot down what's left of your makeup. Cup your hands and splash cool water on your face. Pat dry. Take out your emergency kit and start to patch up for round two. Apply foundation or powder, a touch of blush, add foundation to the lips to allow a fresh lipstick application, and reapply a dressier color from your arsenal, one with a touch of depth or shimmer . . . it will give you that pick-me-up. Repowder over eye makeup, it will even it all out and erase the day's smudges. Now you're ready for the rest of what today brings!

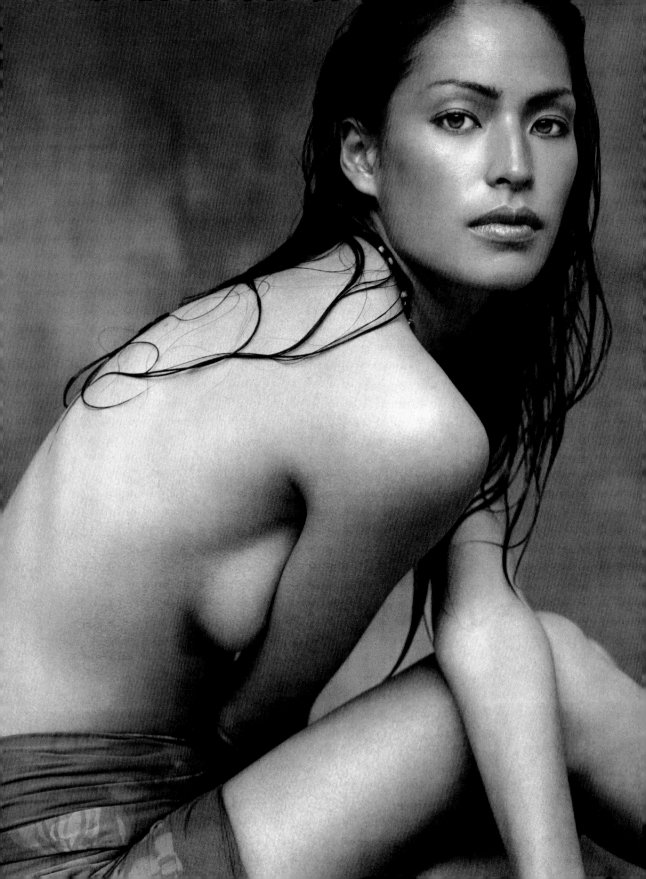

BODY AND SOUL

BEAUTY DOESN'T STOP AT THE FACE. ALL OF YOUR SKIN DESERVES SOME BEAUTY
TREATMENT, STARTING WITH THE FOUR ESSENTIALS: CLEANSING, EXFOLIATING,
MOISTURIZING, AND PROTECTING. BODY PRODUCTS OFTEN COME SCENTED; THE
FRAGRANCE MAY SUFFICE ON ITS OWN OR CAN BE LAYERED WITH SOMETHING ELSE.

Cleansing: Use a nondrying, gentle cleanser. Gels are great and very convenient for
the shower. Unless you really need it, avoid deodorant soaps. Instead, pick
something that smells great and leaves your skin feeling soft.

Exfoliating: A must! Exfoliated skin not only has a special glow, it's softer and silkier to
the touch and absorbs moisturizer better. I also like glycolic washes. I have a big pump
dispenser in my shower for use as needed. You may prefer a loofah, but go gently!

Moisturizing: I prefer lotions, but if you have drier skin, go for a body cream. Apply
to arms, legs, and chest. Your back won't need it because it has more oil glands
than the rest of your body, and hey, you couldn't reach it anyway.

Protecting: I can't say it enough: any skin that's exposed to sun needs to be protected.
Sleeveless tops require sunscreened shoulders and arms. Shorts, miniskirts, and
sandaled feet require sunscreened legs and feet.

SCENT-SATIONAL

Fragrance is one of my favorite topics. I'm passionate about it. For me, scent is part of my lifestyle. Maybe this love of all things scented is in my blood, given my grandmother's profession; I don't know. But to me, scent is an essential indulgence. It sets the tone; it creates a memory. We remember people and homes that smell good. Think of your earliest memories, and, I promise you, a smell will come to mind, be it your grandmother's cooking or your mother's perfume when she was getting ready to go out.

To me, fragrance is a feeling. When I work with my perfumer, I never ask for a specific smell like citrus or rose. I tell her I want "freshness," "warmth," maybe "mystery." My fragrance Trish came about because I was getting ready to go out in a beautiful black dress and I wanted a scent that would capture the feeling of that dress.

Some women have a signature scent that they wear year in, year out. The nice part about that is that the scent becomes your calling card. I love too many scents to choose just one. I like to layer fragrances. Layering lets you create highly personal scents that embrace the moment and your emotions. My fragrance line was conceived with layering in mind. Each scent is pure and simple, able to be worn alone but also ripe for mixing with another. You can also layer by using a differently scented body lotion alongside your perfume. My advice is to experiment and let your nose guide you. You'll know you have made the right choice when the fragrance has lifted your spirits.

THE SCENTED ROOM

Scented candles are one of the most accessible luxuries available. I have scented candles throughout my home and offices. One of the first things I do when I get home—that is, after kicking off my shoes—is to light my candles. The wonderful scents immediately give me that familiar feeling of comfort. Scents set a mood, which is why I put food-inspired aromas in the kitchen and fill the house with season-appropriate scents. In the winter, I love warm spices; in the spring and summer, give me flowers and freshness. Scented candles create an atmosphere that can either uplift or calm you, depending on your needs. Bring one to work and set it on your desk. You'll find people drawn to your office, and my guess is that they won't even know why. Scent has a subtle effect and leaves a lasting impression.

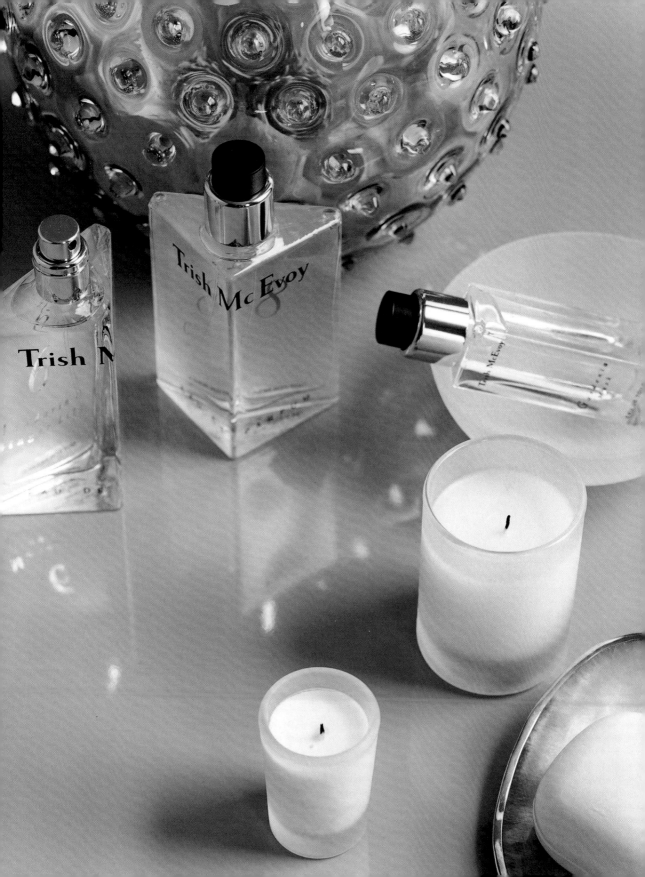

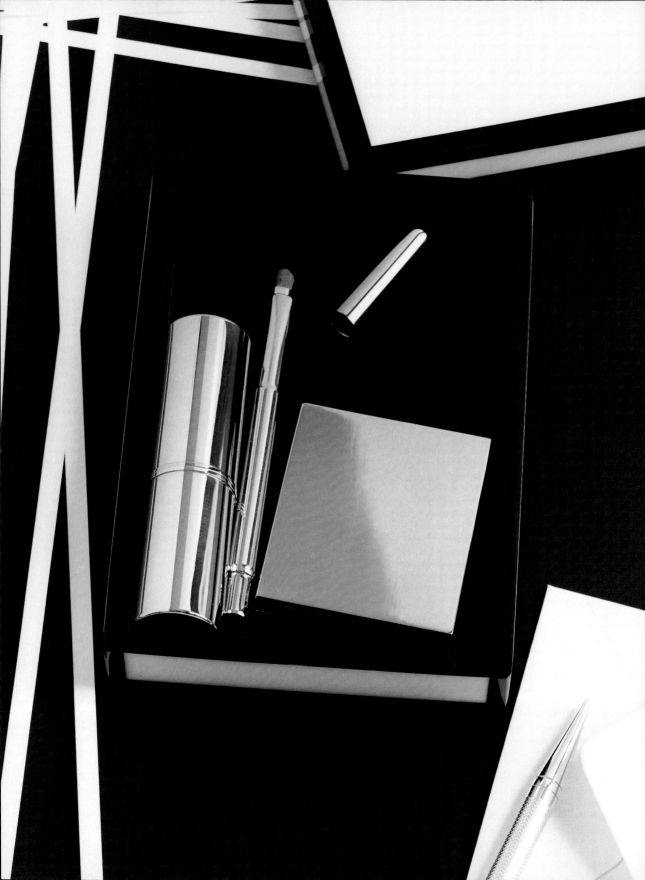

THE GIFT OF BEAUTY

COSMETICS CAN MAKE A WONDERFUL AND PERSONAL GIFT. AS WITH ANY GIFT GIVING, YOU NEED TO THINK ABOUT THE PERSON FOR WHOM YOU'RE BUYING. ONE SIZE DOES NOT FIT ALL ANY MORE THAN IT WOULD IF YOU WERE BUYING A SWEATER AS A GIFT. IF THE WOMAN HAS NEVER SHOWN AN INTEREST IN MAKEUP, YOU'RE NOT ABOUT TO CONVERT HER, BUT YOU MAY CHARM HER WITH A MAKEUP LESSON THAT COULD OPEN HER TO THE POSSIBILITY. SOME GIFT IDEAS TO THINK ABOUT:

A LUXE BRUSH OR BRUSH SET
Many women don't treat themselves to a good brush. When in doubt, pick up a blush brush, the most useful brush of all. If you suspect she has good brushes, then consider a petite brush kit for her handbag or something very special, like a retractable brush with a silver handle that she can carry with her wherever she goes.

A PERSONALIZED GIFT BOX
Have fun and make it up yourself. For example, if she's planning a trip, you can create a "sun package," with SPF protection for face and body, a self-tanner, some lip balm, and a sunny-scented after-sun body lotion. Throw in a pair of goggles. If she's not feeling well, maybe she'd love a body lotion, some bath gel, and a scented candle. Or if she's just tired and overworked, maybe a gift of luxurious treatments.

A MAKEUP KIT
This is a great way for a woman to explore color options. I've created a choice of lip kits, face kits, eye kits, and cheek kits. Play it safe with neutrals or introduce her to a new world of color.

PRODUCTS IN HER FRAGRANCE
Another thoughtful and much-appreciated gift. Go for the indulgent pieces, like body lotions, shower gels, and creams. Or go for smaller-sized fragrances for her purse so that she'll have options, including layering scents together.

A SCENTED CANDLE
Timeless and ageless, whether you know the woman well or not. Perfect for just about any occasion, including as a hostess gift or to say thanks for a job well done. In fact, they're well worth stocking up on to have available for last-minute gift giving.

A PLANNER OR MAKEUP CASE
Either is great, but I suggest you put something in it, even if it's as simple as a lip balm or an eyelash curler. Better yet, add a gift certificate. Now that's a gift of beauty!

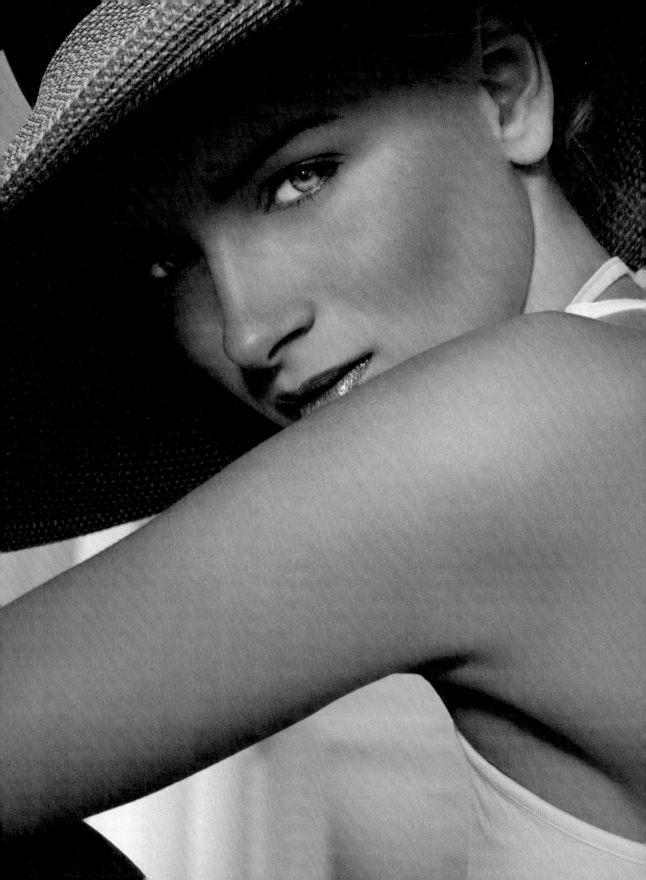

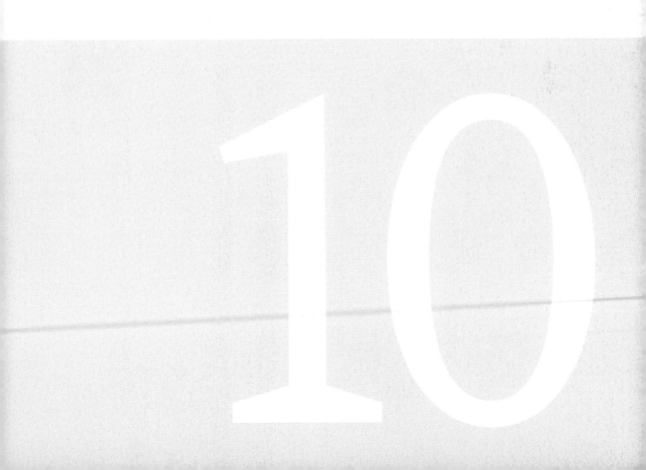

ATTITUDE IS EVERYTHING: *Keeping a Positive Outlook*

THERE ARE DAYS YOU LOOK GREAT AND FEEL CONFIDENT AND THERE ARE DAYS. . . MAKEUP CAN HELP BRIGHTEN YOU UP, AND LITERALLY PUT A FRESH FACE ON THE DAY AHEAD.

I enjoy helping women feel good about their appearance. It empowers women, and I take great joy in that power. The more knowledge I can give you, the better choices you make and the more in control you are of your beauty regimen. You can be more open to new ideas if you understand how they work and what they can do for you. Appearance is a form of self-expression and for many of us a source of confidence. Make no apologies if it takes you an hour to put on your makeup and you enjoy every minute of it. By all means, enhance and beautify what you can. After that, however, get on with your day. Beauty is about style and how you carry yourself. I believe that such beauty is attainable for every woman.

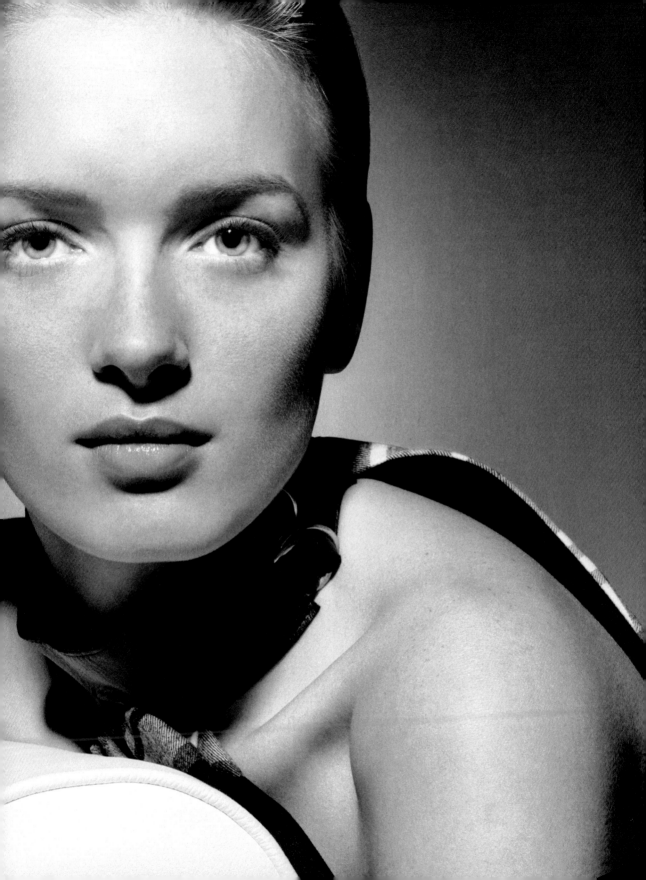

OXOXOX
XOXOXO
OXOXOX

A LIFE OF BEAUTY

My best advice yet: Engage all your senses and indulge in pleasure wherever and however you can. Spend time with your family and friends. Furnish your home with the joy of flowers and music and great food. Literally, stop and smell the roses. Enjoy a sunset. Take a walk. Give yourself the gift of time, and take an hour to do nothing but observe the beauty of nature. Inhale deeply and absorb the moment! Seek new adventures. Find reasons to laugh. Share your love every day. I try not to let a single day go by without telling my husband and all those I love how fortunate I am to have them in my life. Life is a matter of focus, and it is what you decide it will be. Make the most of every experience, and your life will be filled with beauty, I promise.

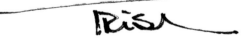

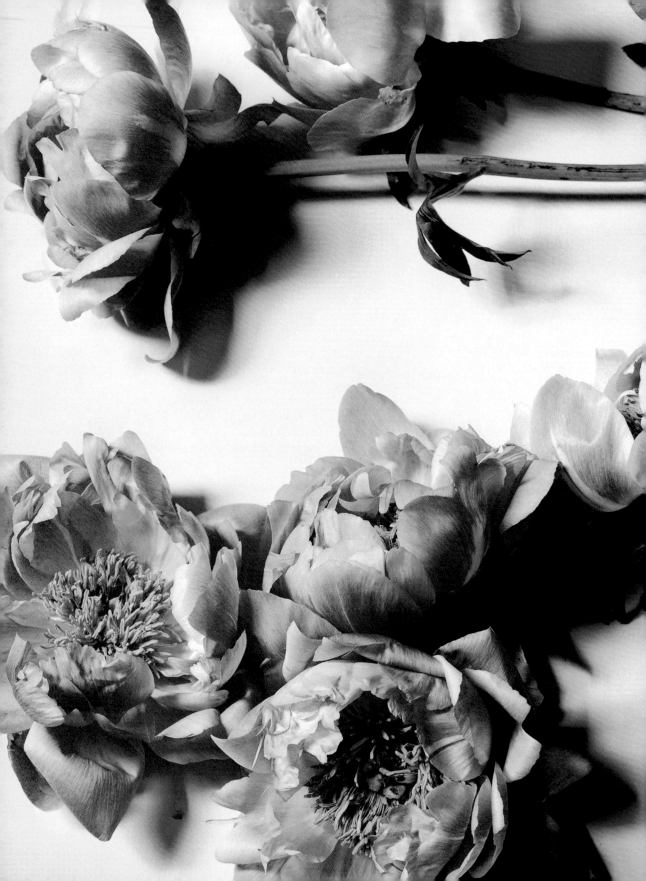

INDEX

CREDITS

front cover: MAKEUP lipstick: paris red PHOTOGRAPHER greg delves *endpapers:* PHOTOGRAPHER greg delves *page 2:* MAKEUP face: weekend/pink blush, foundation tinted moisturizer; eyes: natural, buff, topaz bronzer definer; lips: nude lip liner, sparkling pink sexy gloss FASHION scarf, pucci, available at henri bendel; halter top, ralph lauren; earrings, erwin pearl; bracelet, alexis bittars; PHOTOGRAPHER daniela federici *page 5:* blush, petal eye shadow, dual bronzer, even skin powder, sunkissed powder PHOTOGRAPHER greg delves *page 18:* eye shadow: deep aubergine definer, haze, dew blossom, crystal PHOTOGRAPHER greg delves *page 20:* trish mcevoy portrait PHOTOGRAPHER michel arnaud *page 34:* MAKEUP face: tinted moisturizer, blush natural; eyes: natural waterstix; lips: rosette gloss PHOTOGRAPHER daniela federici *page 40:* MAKEUP face: cheeks easy going blush; lips: cashmere gloss PHOTOGRAPHER daniela federici *page 48:* trish mcevoy planner: luxury orange mini planner, luxury pink mini planner PHOTOGRAPHER greg delves *page 51:* trish mcevoy planner: petite black planner, mini black planner, large black planner PHOTOGRAPHER greg delves *page 54–55:* trish mcevoy planner: luxury mini pink planner PHOTOGRAPHER greg delves *page 56:* trish mcevoy card: maxed out be prepared pink PHOTOGRAPHER greg delves *page 58:* PHOTOGRAPHER greg delves *page 62:* PHOTOGRAPHER martyn thompson *page 64:* PHOTOGRAPHER martyn thompson *page 68:* trish mcevoy mini brushes PHOTOGRAPHER greg delves *page 72:* PHOTOGRAPHER martyn thompson *page 74–75:* trish mcevoy brushes PHOTOGRAPHER greg delves *page 76–77:* trish mcevoy brushes PHOTOGRAPHER greg delves *page 78:* PHOTOGRAPHER martyn thompson *page 81:* lower left and right mirrors, waterworks PHOTOGRAPHER greg delves *page 82:* PHOTOGRAPHER martyn thompson *page 84:* crystal eye shadow, london face shine, warm ginger, satin rose, dual bronzer, sweet dreams lip gloss PHOTOGRAPHER greg delves *page 87:* MAKEUP face: tinted moisturizer, cheek color natural and weekend; lips: lip and cheek stain blush, gloss rosette PHOTOGRAPHER daniela federici *page 89:* MAKEUP face: blush model's choice; eyes: base eye waterstix natural, crease of eye waterstix taupe, eyeliner deep aubergine, highlighter glaze cream; lips:

sparkling ginger, gloss gold rush PHOTOGRAPHER daniela federici *page 90:* MAKEUP face: weekend bronzer, bohemian face shine; eye: copper shimmer and lilac, eyeliner black; lips; sparkling bronze, lip liner cocoa, gloss lucite PHOTOGRAPHER daniela federici *page 93:* MAKEUP face: even skin foundation, even skin powder, pink blush; eyes: warm beige; lips: lip and cheek stain essential pencil sweet berry FASHION necklace, sarah gore reeves PHOTOGRAPHER daniela federici *page 97:* bronze face shine, dual bronzer, malibu face shine, bohemian face shine, pink face shine, london face shine PHOTOGRAPHER greg delves *page 104:* MAKEUP face: tinted moisturizers, london face shine, easy going blush; eyes: topaz waterstix, lilac waterstix, deep aubergine definer; lips: lip and cheek tint, sparkling blush lip color, sexy gloss FASHION dress, alberto ferretti PHOTOGRAPHER daniela federici DOG chloé *page 106:* MAKEUP face: even skin foundation, london bronzer, pink shimmer; eyes: cashmere auburn, sugar glaze, black defined; lips: sparkling nude lip liner 21, gloss cashmere FASHION pink satin top, plein sud, available at henri bendel PHOTOGRAPHER daniela federici *page 111:* MAKEUP face: tinted moisturizer, lip and cheek tint, natural blush; eyes: natural and shell waterstix; lips: lip liner 21, rio lip color, sherry red gloss FASHION necklace, fragments PHOTOGRAPHER daniela federici *page 113:* MAKEUP face: london face shine, tangerine blush; eyes: liner brown, base lid bone, crease of eye ginger; lips: lip liner nude, cheri lip color, luscious gloss PHOTOGRAPHER daniela federici *page 115:* MAKEUP face: cream powder makeup, london face shine, champagne shimmer, easy glowing blush; eyes: cream glaze, warm ginger, black definer, false lashes; lips: nude lip liner, casual lipstick, rosette gloss PHOTOGRAPHER daniela federici *page 122:* MAKEUP face: tinted moisturizer, blush natural; eyes: waterstix natural; lips: rosette gloss FASHION tank top, dkny PHOTOGRAPHER daniela federici *page 125:* MAKEUP face: tinted moisturizer, blush natural; eyes: natural and waterstix; lips: rosette gloss lip liner PHOTOGRAPHER daniela federici *page 126:* MAKEUP face: tinted moisturizer, pink face shine, natural blush; eyes: natural and shell waterstix; lips: nude lip liner, rosette gloss FASHION earrings, baccarat PHOTOGRAPHER daniela federici *page 129:* MAKEUP face: tinted moisturizer, lip and cheek tint, natural blush; eyes, natural and shell waterstix; lips: lip liner 21, rio lip color, sherry red gloss FASHION necklace, fragments PHOTOGRAPHER daniela federici *page 131:* MAKEUP face: even skin foundation, sunkissed all over face color, london and malibu face shine; eyes: waterstix shell natural and topaz bronze lip liner; lips: sparkling pink sexy gloss nude lip liner FASHION choker, max mara PHOTOGRAPHER daniela federici *page 132:* MAKEUP face: shimmer powder champagne, blush pink; eyes: base eyelid natural, crease earth, eyeliner rich brown; lips: almost there, lip liner nude PHOTOGRAPHER daniela federici *page 135:* MAKEUP face: tinted moisturizer, face shine bronzer and pink; eyes: waterstix natural and topaz liner defined; lips: cashmere gloss, lip liner nude PHOTOGRAPHER daniela federici *page 138:* MAKEUP face: face shine london, tangerine blush; eyes: base eye lid bone, crease of eye ginger, eyeliner rich brown; lips: lip color cheri, luscious gloss, lip liner nude PHOTOGRAPHER daniela federici *page 139:* MAKEUP eyes: base eye lid bone, crease of eye taupe, eyeliner rich brown PHOTOGRAPHER daniela federici *page 140:* MAKEUP eyes: base eye lid shaper soft peach and ginger buff, eyeliner deep aubergine PHOTOGRAPHER daniela federici *page 142:* MAKEUP eyes: base eye natural mixes with bronzer, eyeliner bronze definer PHOTOGRAPHER daniela federici *page 148:* MAKEUP face: tinted moisturizer, face shine bronzer and pink; eyes:, waterstix natural and topaz liner defined; lips: cashmere gloss, lip liner nude PHOTOGRAPHER daniela federici *page 150:* MAKEUP face: tinted moisturizer, bronze, london and bohemian face shines; eyes: topaz waterstix, nova definer; lips: sparkling ginger, lip liner nude PHOTOGRAPHER daniela federici *page 153:* MAKEUP face: cream powder makeup, london face shine, champagne shimmer, easy glowing blush; eyes: cream glaze, warm ginger, black definer, false lashes; lips: nude lip liner, casual lipstick, rosette gloss PHOTOGRAPHER daniela federici *page 154:* MAKEUP face: cream powder foundation, nude shimmering powder, london face shine, natural blush; eyes: warm beige, ginger, cashmere, and buff shadows, eyeliner black and finish line, eyeliner nova; lips: sparkling pink, lip liner rio, luxe gloss PHOTOGRAPHER daniela federici

page 157: MAKEUP face: shimmering powder bronze, weekend bronzer, blush bohemian; eyes: base eyelid, 18k and ginger shadow, crease of eye crimson, eyeliner black; lips: sparkling ginger, lip liner angelina jolie, gloss natural PHOTOGRAPHER daniela federici page 158: paris red lipstick PHOTOGRAPHER greg delves page 159: sweet dreams gloss kit PHOTOGRAPHER greg delves page 160: PHOTOGRAPHER daniela federici page 166–167: MAKEUP eyes: natural waterstix, eyeliner bronzer definer PHOTOGRAPHER daniela federici page 171: ice nude lip liner; PHOTOGRAPHER greg delves page 172: MAKEUP face: tinted moisturizer, london and malibu face shine, natural blush; eyes: warm beige, cashmere and brown definer; lips: lip liner deep rosette, lips stain rose, lucite gloss FASHION coat, burberry; bag, suarez PHOTOGRA-PHER daniela federici page 175: face: tinted moisturizer, face shine pink, natural blush; eyes: waterstix natural, shell, and topaz, bronze and nova definer; lips: sparkling blush, nude lip liner, gloss sexy FASHION bikini, benneton; top, pucci; glasses, chanel PHOTOGRAPHER daniela federici page 178: PHO-TOGRAPHER martyn thompson page 181: PHOTOGRAPHER martyn thompson page 183: PHOTOGRAPHER martyn thompson page 186-187: FASHION dress, max mara, available at saks fifth avenue; shoes, christian loubitane, available at saks fifth avenue PHOTOGRAPHER daniela federici page 190: PHOTOGRAPHER daniela federici page 193: FASHION dress, jil sander; earrings, simon alcantara, available at bergdorf goodman PHOTOGRAPHER daniela federici page 198: PHOTOGRAPHER daniela federici page 201: PHO-TOGRAPHER martyn thompson page 202: PHOTOGRAPHER martyn thompson page 204: MAKEUP face: bronze face shine, easy going blush; eyes: natural waterstix, bronzer definer; lips: lip liner nude, sparkling blush, sexy gloss FASHION top, benneton; hat, eric javitz, available at saks fifth avenue PHOTOGRAPHER daniela federici page 207: FASHION top, jil sander PHOTOGRAPHER daniela federici page 210: PHOTOGRAPHER martyn thompson end sheet: PHOTOGRAPHER greg delves back cover: MAKEUP face: tinted moisturizer, lip and cheek tint, natural blush; eyes, natural and shell waterstix; lips: lip liner 21, rio lip color, sherry red gloss FASHION necklace, fragments PHOTOGRAPHER daniela federici page 122: MAKEUP face: tinted moisturizer, blush natural; eyes: waterstix natural; lips: rosette gloss FASHION tank top, dkny PHOTOGRAPHER daniela federici page 125: MAKEUP face: tinted moisturizer, blush natural; eyes: natural and waterstix; lips: rosette gloss lip liner PHOTOGRAPHER daniela federici page 126: MAKEUP face: tinted moisturizer, pink face shine, natural blush; eyes: natural and shell waterstix; lips: nude lip liner, rosette gloss FASHION earrings, baccarat PHOTOGRAPHER daniela federici page 129: MAKEUP face: tinted moisturizer, lip and cheek tint, natural blush; eyes, natural and shell waterstix; lips: lip liner 21, rio lip color, sherry red gloss FASHION necklace, fragments PHOTOGRAPHER daniela federici page 131: MAKEUP face: even skin foundation, sunkissed all over face color, london and malibu face shine; eyes: waterstix shell natural and topaz bronze lip liner; lips: sparkling pink sexy gloss nude lip liner FASHION choker, max mara PHOTOGRAPHER daniela federici page 132: MAKEUP face: shimmer powder champagne, blush pink; eyes: base eyelid natural, crease earth, eyeliner rich brown; lips: almost there, lip liner nude PHOTOGRAPHER daniela federici page 135: MAKEUP face: tinted mois-turizer, face shine bronzer and pink; eyes: waterstix natural and topaz liner defined; lips: cashmere gloss, lip liner nude PHOTOGRAPHER daniela federici page 138: MAKEUP face: face shine london, tangerine blush; eyes: base eye lid bone, crease of eye ginger, eyeliner rich brown; lips: lip color cheri, luscious gloss, lip liner nude PHOTOGRAPHER daniela federici page 139: MAKEUP eyes: base eye lid bone, crease of eye taupe, eyeliner rich brown PHOTOGRAPHER daniela federici page 140: MAKEUP eyes: base eye lid shaper soft peach and ginger buff, eyeliner deep aubergine PHOTOGRAPHER daniela federici page 142: MAKEUP eyes: base eye natural mixes with bronzer, eyeliner bronze definer PHOTOGRAPHER daniela federici page 148: MAKEUP face: tinted moisturizer, face shine bronzer and pink; eyes:, waterstix natural and topaz liner defined; lips: cashmere gloss, lip liner nude PHOTOGRAPHER daniela federici page 150: MAKEUP face: tinted moisturizer, bronze, london and bohemian face shines; eyes: topaz waterstix, nova definer; lips: sparkling ginger, lip liner nude PHOTOGRAPHER daniela federici page 153: MAKEUP face:

cream powder makeup, london face shine, champagne shimmer, easy glowing blush; eyes: cream glaze, warm ginger, black definer, false lashes; lips: nude lip liner, casual lipstick, rosette gloss PHOTOGRAPHER daniela federici *page 154:* MAKEUP face: cream powder foundation, nude shimmering powder, london face shine, natural blush; eyes: warm beige, ginger, cashmere, and buff shadows, eyeliner black and finish line, eyeliner nova; lips: sparkling pink, lip liner rio, luxe gloss PHOTOGRAPHER daniela federici *page 157:* MAKEUP face: shimmering powder bronze, weekend bronzer, blush bohemian; eyes: base eyelid, 18k and ginger shadow, crease of eye crimson, eyeliner black; lips: sparkling ginger, lip liner angelina jolie, gloss natural PHOTOGRAPHER daniela federici *page 158:* paris red lipstick PHOTOGRAPHER greg delves *page 159:* sweet dreams gloss kit PHOTOGRAPHER greg delves *page 160:* PHOTOGRAPHER daniela federici *page 166–167:* MAKEUP eyes: natural waterstix, eyeliner bronzer definer PHOTOGRAPHER daniela federici *page 171:* ice nude lip liner; PHOTOGRAPHER greg delves *page 172:* MAKEUP face: tinted moisturizer, london and malibu face shine, natural blush; eyes: warm beige, cashmere and brown definer; lips: lip liner deep rosette, lips stain rose, lucite gloss FASHION coat, burberry; bag, suarez PHOTOGRA-PHER daniela federici *page 175:* face: tinted moisturizer, face shine pink, natural blush; eyes: waterstix natural, shell, and topaz, bronze and nova definer; lips: sparkling blush, nude lip liner, gloss sexy FASHION bikini, benneton; top, pucci; glasses, chanel PHOTOGRAPHER daniela federici *page 178:* PHO-TOGRAPHER martyn thompson *page 181:* PHOTOGRAPHER martyn thompson *page 183:* PHOTOGRAPHER martyn thompson *page 186-187:* FASHION dress, max mara, available at saks fifth avenue; shoes, christian loubitane, available at saks fifth avenue PHOTOGRAPHER daniela federici *page 190:* PHOTOGRAPHER daniela federici *page 193:* FASHION dress, jil sander; earrings, simon alcantara, available at bergdorf goodman PHOTOGRAPHER daniela federici *page 198:* PHOTOGRAPHER daniela federici *page 201:* PHO-TOGRAPHER martyn thompson *page 202:* PHOTOGRAPHER martyn thompson *page 204:* MAKEUP face: bronze face shine, easy going blush; eyes: natural waterstix, bronzer definer; lips: lip liner nude, sparkling blush, sexy gloss FASHION top, benneton; hat, eric javitz, available at saks fifth avenue PHOTOGRAPHER daniela federici *page 207:* FASHION top, jil sander PHOTOGRAPHER daniela federici *page 210:* PHOTOGRAPHER martyn thompson *end sheet:* PHOTOGRAPHER greg delves *back cover:* MAKEUP face: tinted moisturizer, lip and cheek tint, natural blush; eyes, natural and shell waterstix; lips: lip liner 21, rio lip color, sherry red gloss FASHION necklace, fragments PHOTOGRAPHER daniela federici